K

D0753147

Conducting Research in Long-Term Care Settings

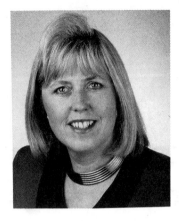

Brenda Lewis Cleary, PhD, RN, FAAN, received a BSN and MSN from Indiana University and a PhD in Nursing from The University of Texas at Austin. She has practiced as a gerontological clinical nurse specialist, in both primary and long-term care settings. Dr. Cleary was a co-investigator on a project entitled, "Management of Problems Associated with Dementia," funded through the National Institute for Nursing Research and the National Institute on Aging. She is a past president of the Alzheimer's Association of Texas and currently serves on the Board of Directors of the Alzheimer's Association, Eastern NC Chapter. She is a Sigma Theta Tau Virginia Henderson fellow as well as a fellow in the American Academy of Nursing. Until July of 1994, Dr. Cleary was Regional Dean and Professor at Texas Tech University Health Sciences Center School of Nursing where she received the Excellence in Teaching Award and the President's Academic Achievement Award. Other honors include the NC Nurses Association Nurse Researcher of the Year Award (1997), distinguished alumna awards from University of Texas at Austin and Indiana University Schools of Nursing, in 1998 and 1999 respectively, and recognition as being among the Great 100 Nurses of North Carolina (2000). She was a 2001 participant in Leadership America and a member of the 2002 cohort of Robert Wood Johnson Executive Nurse Fellows. She currently holds the position of Executive Director of the North Carolina Center for Nursing, a state funded agency committed to assuring nursing resources to meet the health-care needs of the citizens of North Carolina. Dr. Cleary served on the NC Long-Term Care Roundtable and currently serves on the North Carolina Institute of Medicine, both gubernatorial appointments.

Conducting Research in Long-Term Care Settings

Brenda Lewis Cleary, PhD, RN, FAAN

 Springer Publishing Company

Springer Publishing Company, Inc.
536 Broadway
New York, NY 10012-3955

Acquisitions Editor: Ruth Chasek
Production Editor: J. Hurkin-Torres
Cover design by Joanne Honigman

03 04 05 06 07 / 5 4 3 2 1

Library of Congress Cataloging-in-Publication Data

Cleary, Brenda Lewis.
    Conducting research in long-term care settings / Brenda Lewis Cleary.
        p. cm.
    Includes bibliographical references and index.
    ISBN 0-8261-1895-X
    1. Long-term care of the sick—Research. 2. Nursing home care—Research.
3. Long-term care facilities—Research. 4. Aged—Long-term care—Research.
5. Community health services for the aged—Research. I. Title.
    RA644.5.C544 2004
    362.1'6'072—dc21   2004052815

Printed in the United States of America by Maple-Vail Book Manufacturing Group.

This book is dedicated to my family and family of friends, as a tribute to their love and encouragement.

Contents

Preface

A discussion of research in long-term care is a timely topic as we face unprecedented demand for the delivery of long-term care services. Nursing homes, as settings for long-term care and as sociocultural phenomena, are often poorly understood. They are the subject of much scrutiny by the public and much attention, often negative, by the media. Nursing homes, primarily due to regulatory requirements, are rich repositories of data, yet are underutilized for controlled research studies. However, there is growing interest in efforts to improve the quality of care for the high-risk populations that nursing homes serve. Additionally, an increasing number of individuals with long-term care needs are being served at home, providing another setting for long-term care research.

This hands-on guidebook is offered as a tool to help increase research in long-term care settings and both nursing homes and the home setting will be addressed. Furthermore, it is designed to fill a gap in the available literature for graduate students and others interested in the important work of improving the science of long-term care. The first chapter provides the reader with an overview of the characteristics of long-term care in the U.S., including the types of residents/clients served, and the organizational and regulatory context. Chapter 2 deals with the state of the science of long-term care research and addresses common clinical and other issues likely to be of interest to researchers. Health services and health policy research are also addressed. Chapter 3 discusses the ethics of research among subjects who are often vulnerable and cannot speak for themselves. Chapter 4 addresses methodological issues, and Chapters 5 and 6 provide practical guidelines for getting started and implementing a long-term care research project. Chapter 7, the final chapter, provides brief advice regarding research dissemination.

Acknowledgments

I wish to acknowledge Dr. Mary Ann Matteson, who mentored me in the process of gerontological research and in the fine art of authoring. I wish her well in her retirement as she goes on to write books for her grandchildren.

Chapter 1

Long-Term Care
in the United States

The concept of long-term care brings to mind images of chronic illness
and aging, issues of policy and regulation, and concerns about quality,
continuity, and financing. Some definitions are in order. According to a
fact sheet published in 1997 by the National Academy on Aging, *long-term
care* refers to a broad range of services provided to persons who, as the
result of chronic illness or frailty, are unable to function independently
on a daily basis. In other words, these services are designed for persons
requiring assistance with one or more *activities of daily living*. The need
for long-term care may arise from primarily physical limitations (such
as those brought about by heart disease, stroke, respiratory illness, or
musculoskeletal disorders) or from conditions leading to cognitive and/or
mental impairment (such as dementia or other trauma or disease of the
central nervous system, mental illness, or mental retardation). A 1996
report on chronic care in the United States by the University of California
at San Francisco Institute for Health and Aging, and commissioned by the
Robert Wood Johnson Foundation, differentiated the goals of chronic care
from those of acute care: whereas the aim of acute care is to restore a
person to a previous level of function, chronic care seeks to maintain
function, facilitate adjustment, promote independence, and, if possible,
prevent further deterioration.

About 12.8 million Americans, 57 percent of whom are age 65 or over,
report a need for long-term care, and the number is expected to grow
exponentially. By 2020 it is projected that 80 percent of health-care spending in the United States will be related to chronic illness. Problems faced
by the chronically ill and their families include a fragmented and uncoordi-
nated care delivery system, inadequate funding/reimbursement for the ser-

1

vices needed, lack of accommodation for functional limitations, and lost opportunities for a fuller life (Anderson, 2002). Branch (2002) identified the following weak links in the long-term continuum of care: lack of a seamless continuum of care, inadequate information and referral services to guide informal support networks, and lack of professional services to construct and manage the continuum of long-term care.

It is important to remember that most long-term care consists of unreimbursed or informal care provided by family and friends. However, formalized home and community-based services have increased dramatically in the last decade, becoming a $100 billion a year industry, second only to hospitals (Long Term Care Education.com, 2002). Community-based long-term care is delivered in adult day-care centers, senior centers, and through nutrition programs; transportation services, companion services, and telephone reassurance programs are also available (Lieberman, 2000). Long-term care services, including health care and social and assistive services, are also increasingly being delivered in the home. The continuum of care progresses through residential facilities known as assisted living centers or adult care homes to nursing homes. The delivery of long-term care has evolved to follow market demands, ranging from hospital-like subacute care, in which care is complex, but the recipients of care are medically stable, to assisted living or adult care homes, in which residents are able to provide most of their own care, but are offered a secure environment, housekeeping, congregate meals, and assistance with personal care, to nursing facilities, which provide skilled nursing services in Medicare-certified agencies as well as what has traditionally been considered intermediate care which offers comprehensive assistance with activities of daily living, and is funded by Medicaid or private sources. Some adult-care homes are also Medicaid-certified and there are Medicaid waiver programs for a range of community-based services. Continuing care retirement communities offer a range of options from independent living to a continuum of long-term health services (Long Term Care Education.com, 2002). It is likely that the needs of aging baby boomers will be a powerful force in further driving changes in the market for long-term care services (Beck & Chumbler, 1997).

In describing the evolution of long-term care facilities in the United States, Kane (1996) referred to the nursing home as the offspring of the boarding house setting as well as the stepchild of the hospital. The development of the nursing home was fostered by the Social Security Act of 1935, which denied coverage for residents of facilities that were publicly funded or run by city or county governments. The creation of Medicare and

Medicaid in 1965 ushered in the development of the modern-day nursing home. Nursing homes also became part of the landscape of rural United States (Rowles, Beaulieu, & Myers, 1996).

The National Academy on Aging (1997) has projected an exponential increase in the number of elderly persons in need of a nursing home. By the year 2018, an estimated 3.6 million elderly persons will need nursing home care, an increase of more than 2 million from the current figure. More than 57 percent of formal long-term care services are financed through governmental programs, with Medicaid being the primary source of publicly financed long-term care. Medicare was never intended to cover long-term care needs. Cohen (1998) identified emerging trends in long-term care financing, including the increasing role of states as well as individual accountability, and the impact of managed care. He described the development of social health maintenance organizations, which include community care services and short-term nursing home care, chronicling the evolution of the concepts of subacute care and assisted living.

This book focuses on the nursing home as an institutional setting for long-term care and as an important but underused setting for research, but it also provides guidance on the conduct of gerontological research in other long-term care settings, specifically in adult care homes or assisted living facilities, and in home care. Many of the same principles apply in terms of recruiting subjects and methodological and ethical issues. However, investigators interested in conducting research in a nursing home must first be aware of the unique culture of the nursing home environment, an environment influenced by heavy regulation.

CHARACTERISTICS OF U.S. NURSING HOMES

Nursing homes in the United States are either freestanding, part of a retirement or continuing care community, or, less often, affiliated with a hospital. They may be privately owned by an individual or group, or may be part of a small or large corporation or chain of nursing homes. According to the Medical Expenditure Panel Survey (MEPS) Chartbook #3 (Rhoades & Krauss, 1999), nearly two thirds of nursing home facilities are for profit. Just over 26 percent are not for profit, such as facilities owned and operated by religious communities. The remaining 8 percent are owned by local or State governments, or by the Federal government.

The most recent analysis of the MEPS Nursing Home Component (Rhoades & Krauss, 1999) reveals that the number of nursing homes in the United States increased by 19.9 percent from 1987 to 1996. There were 16,840 nursing homes in 1996, for a total of 1.76 million beds, compared with 14,050 in 1987, for a total of 1.48 million beds. However, the overall number of nursing home beds per 1,000 people in the U.S. declined from 141 to 117, representing a 17 percent decrease. But occupancy rates of nursing homes also declined, from 92.3 percent in 1987 to 88.8 percent in 1996, reflecting the fact that long-term care needs are increasingly being met outside of nursing home facilities. The average size of a nursing home remained about the same at approximately 105 beds.

The cost of nursing home care ranges from $33,000–$95,000 a year (Harrington, Carillo, Thollaug, & Summers, 1997). Medicaid, a federal and state need-based medical assistance program available when personal funds are insufficient or depleted, paid for 68–69 percent of nursing home care in 1995, with private payment covering about 23–24 percent. Medicare paid for 8 percent of nursing home care in 1995, up from 5 percent in 1991 (Harrington, Carillo, Thollaug, & Summers, 1997). Medicare, a Federal insurance program for people over 65, and certain disabled people, pays for only limited periods of skilled nursing care following a three-day qualifying stay in a hospital, i.e., a maximum of 100 days, governed by utilization review procedures, and only in Medicare-certified facilities. The number of Medicare-certified nursing homes is growing rapidly, a change ushered in by revised certification requirements mandated by federal nursing home reform legislation, the Omnibus Budget Reconciliation Act (OBRA) of 1987. During the period 1987–1996, the proportion of nursing home facilities with Medicare beds increased from 28 to 73 percent (Rhoades & Krauss, 1999). This change also corresponds with increased requirements for skilled care by residents who are older and sicker.

Another emerging phenomenon is the special care unit concept. Almost one fifth of all U.S. nursing homes had at least one special care unit as of 1996. By far the largest type of special care unit is dedicated to specialized Alzheimer's care; 12.6 percent of nursing homes had such units in 1996. Almost 5 percent had distinct rehabilitation or subacute units. Another 5 percent had a ventilator unit or other type of special care unit, including hospice, HIV/AIDS, and brain injury units (Rhoades & Krauss, 1999). Special care units, for the most part, employ a philosophy of supportive and palliative care, with comfort and quality of life taking priority over life-prolonging interventions (Johnston & Reifler, 1999).

The Balanced Budget Act of 1997 included a mandate that a prospective payment system for both nursing homes and home care be phased in over a three-year period, with nursing homes beginning the process on July

1, 1998. Nursing homes across the country are implementing case-mix adjustment and navigating a prospective payment system (PPS), which replaces the previous cost-based system. In nursing homes, case mix is determined through a classification system known as resource utilization groups (RUGs) (Baker, 2000; Mueller, 2000).

Prospective, as opposed to retrospective, payment for health services is certainly not a new concept, having been in place in acute care settings for many years. However, the prospective mechanism of reimbursement and predetermined fixed costs have created a period of instability in terms of financing long-term care, including home and institutional services.

Before the implementation of PPS, Medicare Part A reimbursement for skilled nursing facilities was cost based, with few incentives for savings. Currently, under the Medicare PPS, nursing home facilities are paid a predetermined daily rate for each Medicare recipient. As with other capitated or prospective reimbursement systems, the incentive is to keep costs as low as possible. A facility's case mix is determined from information included in the Minimum Data Set, which will be discussed in detail in the following section of this chapter. RUG methodology is then used to identify levels of care required and determine Medicare coverage eligibility.

According to Krauss and colleagues (1997) of the Agency for Healthcare Research and Quality (AHRQ), the proportion of nursing home facilities owned or leased by nursing home chains is increasing, and the majority of nursing home facilities are proprietary. Of the approximately 16,800 nursing homes in the United States in 1996, 66 percent operated for profit, and about 68 percent of these for-profit facilities were part of a chain. Not-for-profit homes account for approximately 26 percent of nursing homes, and government-owned facilities make up about 7 percent. While there have historically been few demonstrable differences in for-profit and not-for-profit facilities, Aaronson, Zinn, and Rosko (1994) presented evidence that not-for-profit homes had better staffing and demonstrated better outcomes for residents at high risk. Not-for-profit homes were more likely to increase efficiency in response to environmental pressures, whereas for-profit facilities tended to operate at a high level of efficiency irrespective of environmental or regulatory pressures (Rosko, Chilingerian, Zinn, & Aaronson, 1995).

Kane (1996b) described the nursing home as the backbone of long-term care. He identified several major, interrelated themes that affect nursing home care:

- managed care and changing systems of payment
- diversification

- linkages between acute care and chronic care
- information technology
- evolving ethics
- increasing accountability

The Agency for Healthcare Research and Quality, through its Medical Expenditure Panel Survey (MEPS), is an excellent and growing resource for information on long-term care financing and the characteristics of nursing home facilities. MEPS findings can be obtained at *www.meps. ahrq.gov.*

ORGANIZATIONAL CLIMATE AND CULTURE

The culture of nursing homes is typically influenced by constraints on resources. This is especially true of nursing homes with a large percentage of Medicaid beds, often owing to inadequate reimbursement from Medicaid. Most nursing homes try to create a home-like and supportive environment for residents, while adhering to regulatory structures and processes, and dealing with cost constraints.

In 1998, Bond and Fiedler, using case study methodology, identified broad characteristics of organizational culture in a nursing home:

- treatment of staff members
- effectiveness of leaders in promoting organizational values and philosophy
- staff performance in reflecting the core values of dignity, privacy, choice, and independence for residents
- the organization's mission in terms of the larger environment
- quality of care

Mattiasson and Andersson (1995), in their report on a Swedish study of thirteen nursing homes, found that an organizational climate that staff perceived as creative supported residents' autonomy. The climate was influenced more by the experience of the staff than by the actual workload. Canadian researchers Goodridge and Hack (1996) used a cultural-assessment survey to analyze the culture of the nursing department at a very large (320-bed) long-term care facility. Empathy for residents and concern for their comfort emerged consistently as core values.

It is difficult for nursing homes to maintain an atmosphere that is orderly, calm, and serene. To a great extent, this difficulty is due to the large percentage of residents with some sort of dementia. The nursing home environment is often affected by what may be considered socially inappropriate behavior, including verbal and physical outbursts, public displays of sexual behavior, wandering and pacing, and screaming or moaning. Immobility and incontinence are commonplace. At the same time, nursing homes are typically filled with love and laughter and are generally places where hugs and other displays of affection abound.

One of the most in-depth analyses of everyday life in a nursing home stemmed from the work of Jaber Gubrium in the 1970s. Gubrium examined the social organization of a nursing home by spending several months as a participant-observer. Gubrium's original ethnography was published in 1975, with a later edition published in 1997. In the 1997 edition, Gubrium discussed noteworthy changes in long-term care since his original fieldwork, noting higher acuity and special care units. He also cited rising costs and the emergence of comprehensive assessment systems.

A case study of two nursing home residents by Cleary (1992) yielded information about positive adjustment to nursing home life, including transition, as well as maintenance, in which the nursing home was viewed as a support system. Negative perceptions included a "narrowing" of the residents' worlds, the degree of regimentation, and disruptive behaviors of residents. In a study of 58 nursing home residents, Johnson, Stone, Altmaier, and Berdahl (1998) found that demographic factors did not predict successful adjustment to a nursing home; perceived self-efficacy was a better predictor than locus of control or the degree to which life events are judged to be internally versus externally mediated.

Fitch (1990) proposed a paradigm for nursing home care (the nursing home as neighborhood) and a shift from "providing" care to "facilitating" care. Fitch addressed the unfortunate phenomenon that nursing homes in the United States have come to be perceived as a social problem. Contemporary, holistic approaches to nursing home care include the Eden Alternative, created by William Thomas (1996). The Eden Alternative seeks to create a human habitat infused with life in the form of plants, animals, and children. It involves a multifaceted approach that encourages elders to be an integral part of creating and maintaining the human habitat as a caring community (Klauber, 2000). According to Bruck (1997), more than 100 nursing home facilities in Alabama, Missouri, New York, North Carolina, and Texas have undertaken the challenge of creating such a habitat, with other facilities in Michigan, Minnesota, Nebraska, and South Carolina following suit in the transformation to "Edenized" facilities. Kari and Michel's (1991) Lazarus Project was designed to transform nursing homes through a model of democratic governance that empowers both those who work and those who live in a nursing home facility.

A study published by Castle and Banaszak-Holl (1997) described management team characteristics and innovation in nursing homes. Tenure, educational background, and professional involvement of the top management staff, including 237 directors of nursing and 236 nursing home administrators at 248 facilities, were important factors in explaining the likelihood of innovation. For the purposes of the Castle and Banaszak-Holl study, innovation was operationally defined as computerization of the Minimum Data Set (MDS). Anderson and McDaniel (1998) examined the involvement of RNs in management decisions and found that their primary role was "raising issues," whereas the decision-making activity of "choosing alternatives" often reflected inadequate involvement of the RN staff.

The climate of most nursing homes is affected by outside influences such as corporate policy and culture in the case of nursing home chains. Most nursing homes pay for membership in industry trade associations organized at state and national levels. The American Health Care Association (AHCA) is one of two national trade associations representing the nursing home industry comprises affiliate organizations in each state and the District of Columbia. AHCA affiliate member providers are primarily for-profit nursing homes; the American Association of Homes for the Aging (AAHA) typically represents not-for-profit nursing homes.

THE REGULATORY ENVIRONMENT IN NURSING HOMES

The major goals of long-term care regulation include consumer protection and assuring accountability for publicly funded care. The nursing home industry is the most regulated sector of health care today because of a mandatory licensing and review process; some facilities also choose to apply for accreditation through accrediting agencies such as the Joint Commission on Accreditation of Health Care Organizations (JCAHO). Adherence to mandatory regulations is assessed through annual on-site surveys. Regulators may also make periodic site visits to investigate complaints. When a nursing home facility fails to meet standards of care, as evaluated by state surveyors, a deficiency or citation is issued for each standard violated. Deficiencies vary in weight or severity and in associated penalties. The top ten deficiencies as identified through data from the On-line Survey Certification and Reporting System (OSCAR), a federal online database containing information from more than 16,000 nursing homes in the United States, were:

1. failure to conduct comprehensive resident assessments
2. failure to ensure sanitary food
3. failure to prepare comprehensive resident care plans
4. failure to provide care that protects residents' dignity
5. failure to remove accident hazards
6. inappropriate use of physical restraints
7. inadequate prevention and treatment of pressure ulcers
8. substandard housekeeping
9. failure to accommodate residents' needs
10. substandard infection control

Nursing homes frequently receive negative attention in the media. The public's attention is captured by stories of abuse and neglect of residents because many people perceive residents of nursing homes to be our most vulnerable citizens. In 1986, the Institute of Medicine study on nursing home regulation reported that there were widespread problems in the quality of care and recommended further strengthening of federal regulations for nursing homes. Even though regulatory functions and monitoring are carried out by state departments of health, the nursing home reform legislation passed by Congress in the 1987 Omnibus Budget Reconciliation Act (OBRA) had sweeping regulatory implications. OBRA was implemented by the Health Care Financing Administration (HCFA) of the U.S. Public Health Service in 1990. Among the major mandates of OBRA was the requirement for comprehensive assessments of all nursing home residents (note the use of the term *residents* as opposed to *patients*) to determine their functional and cognitive levels and to generate assessment data to be used in the care-planning process.

OBRA focused on attaining and maintaining the highest mental and physical functional status among residents by improving outcomes in areas such as immobility, incontinence, and pressure ulcers. OBRA also addressed residents' rights, staffing requirements, and other factors associated with delivering long-term care in institutional settings, including reduction of restraints, both chemical and physical, and required preadmission screening of residents for psychiatric illness.

The resident assessment system developed in response to OBRA regulations is a Resident Assessment Instrument (RAI) that contains two key parts. The Minimum Data Set (MDS) is an evolving instrument that has the core elements of comprehensive assessment with triggers to identify areas for in-depth assessment, involving resident assessment protocols (RAPs). The RAPs address delirium, dementia, visual function, communication, activities of daily living, urinary incontinence, psychosocial well-being, mood state, behavioral symptoms, activities, falls, nutritional status, feeding tubes, dehydration, adult safety, fluid maintenance, dental care, pressure ulcers, use of psychotropic drugs, and physical restraints. Individualized care planning for each resident occurs within an interdisciplinary team approach.

The first version of the MDS was launched in 1990, and a revised version (MDS+) was released in 1992. In 1995, MDS 2.0 was unveiled, with a plan for nationwide implementation in 1997 along with a mandate for computerization. The instrument is considered a work in progress (Brooks, 1996). The MDS was developed as an assessment tool that is being refined into a measurement instrument capable of providing accurate and reproducible data. According to Fries (1997), there is growing interest in not only the assessment process, but also the technology of assessment and innovative uses of the data. Innovation also includes adaptation of the instrument for use in a continuum of long-term care settings. The MDS has demonstrated improved reliability estimates over time, with revision of items in the instrument and the addition of new items (Hawes et al., 1995; Morris et al., 1997a). Table 1.1 is a timeline of the development of the MDS. Further information, including the most current version of the instrument, may be obtained through the Centers for Medicare & Medicaid Services at *www.medicare.gov*.

TABLE 1.1   Timeline of the Development of the Minimum Data Set

1959	Senate subcommittee raises concerns about nursing home care quality
1974	Resident assessments required (nonstandardized)
1970s/early 1980s	Ensuring regulatory standards accepted as a responsibility of the Secretary of Health and Human Services
1986	Institute of Medicine study recommends reforming the survey process and requiring standardized resident assessments
1987	OBRA incorporates Institute of Medicine regulations into federal law
1990	Health Care Financing Administration unveils first version of MDS
1992	Health Care Financing Administration launches MDS+
1995–1996	Unveiling and beta testing of MDS 2.0
1997–1998	Implementation and target for computerization of MDS 2.0
2000	Other versions of MDS emerging, such as MDS-HC (Home Care)

In two separate analyses, Marek, Rantz, Fagin, and Wessel Krejci (1996a, 1996b) reported the results of an examination of the progress in nursing home quality since the passage and implementation of OBRA. Based on interviews with 132 professional and support staff members (as well as 59 residents) in six states, the investigators viewed changes brought about by OBRA as positive among all respondents with regard to important quality-of-care issues (e.g., resident assessment, resident rights and dignity, and use of restraints). They raised concern regarding the Preadmission Screening and Resident Review (PASARR) and recommended that the implementation of this tool for screening for psychiatric symptomatology be re-examined (Marek, Rantz, Fagin, & Wessel Krejci, 1996a). Questions about staffing and quality of care in nursing homes posed by Marek, Rantz, Fagin, and Wessel Krejci (1996b) revealed divergent views regarding the impact of OBRA, with most respondents indicating no change or no opinion. The investigators concluded that, while both staffing and overall quality have improved, the improvements may not be adequate. A 2001 report by the Institute of Medicine broadly explored the means for assessing and improving the quality of long-term care and the pragmatic and policy-related challenges of achieving consistent quality across care settings. According to the report, the quality of care, and to a lesser degree, the quality of life in nursing homes have improved since the implementation of OBRA in 1987, even though care is more complex. For example, the use of both physical and chemical restraints has been reduced. However, pain, pressure ulcers, malnutrition, and urinary incontinence continue to be serious challenges in the nursing home population.

CHARACTERISTICS OF NURSING HOME RESIDENTS

Some 2.4 million Americans are institutionalized and reside primarily in nursing homes or in intermediate-care facilities for mentally retarded persons. About two-thirds of the institutionalized population is age 65 or over and the mean age has increased from 83.5 years in 1987 to 84.6 years in 1996 (Rhoades & Krauss, 1999). Age is a definite risk factor for institutionalization: the lifetime risk of spending some time in a nursing home is estimated to be about 39 percent at age 65, but increases to approximately 49 percent by age 85. Owing to the greater likelihood of wives surviving their husbands, women are more likely than men to enter a nursing home; in fact, women make up about 72 percent of the nursing home population (Giacalone, 2001). It is projected that 25 percent of the women who turned age 65 in 1990 will spend 5 or more years in a nursing home, compared with 15 percent of the men who reached age 65 in that same year (National Academy on Aging, 1997). Projections according to a study by Lindrooth, Hoerger, and Norton (2000) sponsored by the Agency for Healthcare Research and Quality (AHRQ) indicated that a 75-year-old in good health has only a 6 percent chance of entering a nursing home by age 80. For 75-year-olds with declining health, the probability increases from 17 percent to 44 percent when cognitive impairment is present. Interestingly, elders' expectations about entering a nursing home turn out to be reasonably close to actual probability. In a study published in 1997, Murtaugh, Kemper, Spillman, and Carson estimated the overall lifetime use of nursing home care to be approximately one year, although Giacalone noted that lengths of stay tend to assume a bimodal distribution, as nursing homes also provide care to people with postacute conditions, with length of stay varying significantly according to diagnosis.

Nursing homes are filled with people who have one (and usually more) chronic illnesses, and increasingly with acutely ill people as well. Decreasing lengths of hospital stay and a rapid shift toward delivering care outside the hospital are trends that at least partly explain the phenomenon of sicker residents in nursing homes. Many hospitals have developed their own subacute care units (Griffin, 1995) to provide extended care that is typically reimbursed by Medicare.

A 1995 profile of nursing home residents revealed that 47–48 percent were chair-bound and nearly 8 percent bedfast, with a high need for assistance with activities of daily living such as eating, dressing, and toileting (Harrington, Carrillo, Thollaug, & Summers, 1997). Krauss and colleagues (1997) noted that nursing home residents have a high degree of functional difficulty, with 83 percent requiring assistance with three or more activities of daily living such as bathing, eating, and toileting.

There are persistent effects of race/ethnicity on the use of nursing homes: nursing home populations are predominately white (nearly 90 percent) and not in parity with the general population (Wallace, Levy-Storms, Kingston, & Andersen, 1998). Chronicity has long been associated with the need for nursing home care, but acuity is also increasing in nursing home facilities (Kane & Kane, 1995). Relatively common problems among nursing home residents include accidental injury and the associated use of physical restraints or psychotropic drugs, pressure ulcers, and incontinence. Primarily due to the high prevalence of dementia, more than half of nursing home residents exhibit behavior disturbances including delusions/hallucinations, aggressive behaviors, stealing and hoarding behaviors, wandering, and dangerous behaviors (Jackson, Spector, & Rabins, 1997). However, according to the 1999 MEPS report, there has actually been a decline in inappropriate and potentially dangerous behavior. It is noteworthy that up to 94 percent of nursing home facilities have organized groups for addressing residents' and families' concerns (Harrington, Carrillo, Thollaug, & Summers, 1997).

STAFFING IN NURSING HOMES

Nursing homes have a nursing home administrator, the chief executive officer, who answers to the owner, board of directors, or other corporate governance structure; credentialing requirements for administrators are regulated at the state level. Nursing homes also include social work and activity staff, and dietary, pharmacy, and rehabilitation services. Of course, the bulk of clinical services is provided by the nursing department under the direction of a Director of Nursing Services. (See Table 1.2.) OSCAR contains important data regarding staffing in nursing homes. According to information derived from the OSCAR database in 1999, AHCA created a sourcebook that illustrated that in an average 110-bed facility, there were a total of 55 direct care nursing staff: 36 certified nursing assistants or nurse aides (NAs), 12 licensed practical nurses (LPNs), and 7 registered nurses (RNs). The number of hours of care by an RN per resident day averaged 0.4, while the licensed practical/vocational nurse (LPN/LVN) hours per resident day averaged 0.7. Nurse assistant (NA) hours averaged 2.3 per resident day. A specific change in staffing requirements for nursing homes instituted by OBRA was the mandate for licensed nurse coverage 24 hours a day and RN coverage at least 8 hours a day, seven days a week. However, because of the nursing shortage at the time of the implementation of OBRA, states were empowered to issue waivers, lessening the potential impact of new staffing requirements on the quality of care. In the years since the implementation of OBRA, there has been a steady decline in the number of waivers granted.

There is a positive relationship between nursing staff levels and the quality of care (Anderson, Hsieh, & Su, 1998; Bliesmer, Smayling, Kane, & Shannon, 1998; Kovner & Harrington, 2001). The Institute of Medicine, in the 1996 landmark report on nursing staff in hospitals and nursing homes, recommended 24-hour RN coverage and the inclusion of advanced-practice RNs (geriatric/gerontological clinical nurse specialists and geriatric nurse practitioners) in both leadership and direct care positions. To further

TABLE 1.2   Nursing Home Staff Members

A typical employee roster:
    licensed nursing home administrator
    director of nursing, a registered nurse
    other registered nurses, including perhaps an assistant director of nursing and an
        inservice educator
    licensed practical or vocational nurses
    certified nursing assistants
    social worker
    activities director
    dietary supervisor and employees
    maintenance worker(s)

Other roles (may be contractual or consultative) include:
    medical director
    advanced practice nurse or physician assistant
    physical therapist, occupational therapist, and other rehabilitation therapists
    pharmacist
    dietician
    beautician/barber

address recommendations regarding minimum staffing standards, a panel of experts was convened by the John A. Hartford Institute for Geriatric Nursing in April 1998. The equivalent of one full-time RN was recommended for every five residents on the day shift, with a ratio of 1:10 evenings and 1:15 nights. Recommended LPN/LVN-to-resident ratios are as follows: 1:15 days, 1:20 evenings, and 1:30 nights (Hartford Institute for Geriatric Nursing, 1999). Nursing homes throughout the country typically fall far short of these staffing recommendations, particularly for registered nurses.

As of 1998, of the more than 1 million caregivers practicing in long-term care facilities, 64.5 percent were NAs, 18.6 percent were LPNs, 14.2 percent were RNs, and 2.8 percent were physical therapists or social workers (Wunderlich & Kohler, 2001). Based on these numbers, it is not surprising that most of the direct care in nursing homes is provided by NAs. OBRA requirements called for greater consistency in the training and testing of NAs for competency within four months of employment. According to a 1995 analysis by Crown, Ahlburg, and MacAdam, NAs are predominately female and three-fourths have not completed high school. They often come from low-income families and earn close to minimum wage, with limited benefits. With the added element of physically and mentally demanding workloads, it is no surprise that their turnover is high. Nursing homes with higher NA ratios, in which NAs' contributions are acknowledged and NAs are embraced as part of the care team, enjoy lower turnover rates (Mor, 1995). However, in a 2000 report, the National Committee to Preserve Social Security and Medicare raised concerns that LPNs, with only one year of training, are often left in charge of nursing home units, leaving NAs without appropriate management and supervision.

The continuity of care may well be affected by high rates of staff turnover. The recruitment and retention of nurses requires progressive practice models and an improved public/professional image (Robertson & Cummings, 1996). It has been shown that the involvement of all levels of staff in interdisciplinary care planning reduces turnover, especially among NAs (Banaszak-Holl & Hines, 1996). The involvement of NAs in shift reports as well as the frequency of unit staff meetings and administrative autonomy in decision making were process variables identified to be significant factors of perceived staff influence in a study of 51 nursing homes by Kruzich (1995).

A 2001 AHCA report addressing staffing for nursing services in U.S. nursing homes indicated vacancies in over 100,000 direct-care nursing positions, including over 65,000 NA positions, 24,000 LPN positions, and 16,000 RN positions. The projected demand for all nursing personnel is expected to increase by 66 to 71.5 percent by 2020. A 2001 report of the Centers for Medicare and Medicaid Services (formerly the Health Care Financing Administration) seeks to expand OBRA '87 staffing requirements to create more specific federal standards for staffing requirements and staffing ratios in the nursing home industry.

The medical care of residents is reviewed at regular intervals (usually every 60 days for long-staying residents) by the resident's physician, physician assistant, or advanced practice nurse. Typically, one physician is hired as the Medical Director. Arrangements are made for specialty care and vision and dental care. Evans and colleagues (1995) presented an overview of the challenges of providing medical care to nursing home residents, especially noting cognitive and functional impairment, polypharmacy (multiple prescription medications), falls, and resistant infections.

QUALITY OF CARE

The term quality implies not only adherence to a set of standards, but ultimately involves a high level of service and customer satisfaction. Three approaches are used for assuring quality of care as well as quality of life, according to a 2001 report by the Institute of Medicine: (1) government and accrediting agency standards along with quality improvement incentives through Medicare, Medicaid, and other payers; (2) consumer choice and market competition; and (3) professional and organizational commitment to quality improvement (Wunderlich & Kohler, 2001). The classic model for evaluating quality, developed by Donabedian (1966), consists of structure, process, and outcomes. It is a useful framework for better understanding the work of nursing homes. Ramsay, Sainfort, and Zimmerman (1995) touted an empirical causal model of structure, process, and outcome dimensions as a first step in managing the quality of nursing home facilities. Further development of the model was accompanied by words of caution because of exogenous factors such as ownership at work in influencing the quality of nursing homes.

Table 1.3 provides specific examples of structural, process, and outcome variables in nursing home settings. *Structural* variables include facility characteristics and organizational structure, staff mix, and resident characteristics or the case mix and payer mix of residents. *Process* variables refer to the actual delivery of services within the context of basic rights and expectations afforded to residents. *Outcomes* and *outcome measures* have become buzzwords and nursing homes are moving toward an outcomes orientation and the expectation of evidenced-based care. The outcomes of nursing home care include the health status and quality of life of residents and the satisfaction of both residents and their families. However, improved health status, especially in terms of biophysical indicators, is not always a realistic expectation of long-term care.

Continuous quality improvement is a data-driven process for improving performance. Principles are derived from a variety of quality pioneers including W. Edwards Demming, Joseph M. Juran, Phillip Joiner, and Brian Joiner. Demming's philosophy and his 14-point approach to achieving quality, which seeks to develop a constancy of purpose, promotes training and leadership, and drives out fear, while avoiding being driven solely by the bottom line, is the most widely applied. The Health Care Financing Administration (HCFA), now the Center for Medicare and Medicaid Services, instituted changes to the State Operations Manual that require surveyors to assess quality indicators such as prevalence of incontinence or multiple medication use. Information obtained through the Minimum Data Set alerts surveyors to possible areas of concerns (Opus Communications, 2000).

In their book on the quality of care in nursing homes, Morris, Lipsitz, Murray, and Belleville-Taylor (1997b) addressed primarily process mea-

TABLE 1.3   Structure, Process, and Outcomes

Structural Measures
  Staffing levels (nurses, PTs, OTs, etc.)
  Staffing mix
  Staff turnover
  Wages/benefits
  Management/leadership structure
  Facility: size, location, ownership
  Availability of private rooms
  Volunteers
  Governance
  Age/condition of plant equipment (includes mobility development)
  Payer mix (percentage of mix, etc.)
  Case mix
  Accreditation
  Teaching status

Process-of-Care Measures
  Assistance with ADL/IADL (includes bathing, skin care)
  Injury (residents and staff)
  Infection control (residents and staff)
  Resident services: special care to prevent problems
  Overuse of restraints
  Use of urinary catheters
  Bladder training
  Delivery of "hotel" services (sanitation)
  Assessment (includes care planning), frequency and completeness
  Prevention of abuse
  Quality assurance (RA and MDS)
  Access to and use of medical care
  Resident rights

Outcome Measures
  Mortality
  Hospitalization
  Facility-acquired pressure sores, skin breakdown
  Change in functional status
  Pain control
  Depression
  Injuries
  Urinary incontinence
  Weight loss
  Infectious disease
  Resident satisfaction
  Family satisfaction
  Thefts/abuse
  Staff injuries/illness
  Staff satisfaction

Source: Wunderlich, Sloan, & Davis, 1996, Table 6.1, p. 130. Reprinted with permission.
Note: ADL = activities of daily living; IADL = instrumental activities of daily living; OT = occupational therapist; PT = physical therapist; RA = resident assessment; MDS = Minimum Data Set.

sures for a host of common problems among chronically ill residents. Problems ranged from physical ailments (such as infections, falls, skin disorders, malnutrition, dehydration, and incontinence, as well as iatrogenic factors associated with polypharmacy) to cognitive, emotional, and behavioral issues. Quality-of-care issues will be addressed extensively in Chapter 2, since tracking outcomes of care and measurement of quality is taking on greater emphasis in nursing homes, consistent with overall trends in the health-care delivery system.

CHARACTERISTICS OF COMMUNITY BASED LONG-TERM CARE

Home health care has been a fast growing industry for the delivery of transitional care (Katz, Kane, & Mezey, 1999), but under Medicaid waivers and demonstration projects, the home is also a more common site for long-term care. Kane, Kane, and Ladd (1998) referred to home care and personal assistant services as the most important building blocks in community-based long-term care. They described the goals of home-based long-term care as consistent with other settings, i.e., maintaining or improving function, enhancing health, minimizing discomfort, and promoting psychosocial well-being while, at the same time, allowing the recipient of care to maintain a connection with family and community. Six kinds of services were identified, including (1) personal assistance with activities of daily living such as bathing, dressing, toileting, and eating; (2) assistance with instrumental activities of daily living, i.e., housekeeping, cooking, laundry, and other chores; (3) nursing services such as monitoring and treatments, including medication assistance; (4) supervision and oversight; (5) rehabilitation services; and (6) case management. Long-term care provided in the home can be broadly grouped into five categories: rehabilitation, convalescent care, ongoing care, hospice care, and respite care. Health services provided include nutritional care, social work, laboratory tests and x-rays, pharmacy services, dental, optical, and podiatric care, and equipment and supplies (National Association for Home Care, 2002). Care may be therapeutic in terms of actually improving health status, or compensatory in helping the patient and family manage a chronic illness or disability.

Modern home care began in England in 1859, when Florence Nightingale assisted William Rathbone in developing a school to train visiting nurses for the purpose of caring for poor sick people in their homes. The influx of poor immigrants with serious health problems to the United States in the late 1800s prompted the philanthropic establishment of visiting nurse services in Boston, Buffalo, New York, and Philadelphia. As these services spread, sliding scale fees were assessed. Visiting Nurses Associations (VNAs) developed as free-standing, not-for-profit agencies across the country. Today, there are also free-standing proprietary as well as hospital-based home care agencies. In addition, some public health agencies provide home visits (Stackhouse, 1998).

Stanhope and Knollmueller (2000) describe several phases of a home-care visit, including the initial contact and previsit activities, through the actual delivery of care, to termination and follow-up. The process of home care typically involves a family and individual assessment, an environmental assessment, a cultural assessment, and a functional assessment.

The hospice movement, with its philosophy of supportive care for patients whose life expectancy is measured in weeks or months, has resulted in hospice becoming an important benefit, supported by both Medicare and private insurance, of the home care landscape. The movement began in 1967 at St. Christopher's Hospice in London. Hospice services in the U.S. center around home care, although services are also provided in hospitals and nursing homes. Hospice providers, recognizing that death is the final stage of life, seek to provide comfort and enhance quality of life for terminally ill patients at home, where they are surrounded by loved ones. Hospice care offers comprehensive palliative treatment (treatment aimed at symptom management as opposed to curing illness) and includes social, emotional, and spiritual services. Hospice services are delivered by an interdisciplinary team, composed primarily of physicians, nurses, social workers, chaplains, professionals, and volunteers. Children as well as adults receive hospice care, but just as with other home-care services, recipients tend to be primarily older people. The National Hospice Organization as well as the National Association for Home Care provide guidance for agencies and clinicians providing hospice care (National Association for Home Care, 2002).

THE REGULATORY AND REIMBURSEMENT ENVIRONMENT

The majority of states require licensure for home care agencies; any agency seeking Medicare certification must be licensed in the state in which it is located, and periodic satisfactory surveys must be conducted to maintain certification. Home-care agencies may also seek voluntary accreditation through the Joint Commission on Accreditation of Healthcare Organizations or the Community Health Accreditation Program. The most common source of reimbursement is Medicare, recently transitioned to a prospective payment scheme. Other payment sources include Medicaid and private insurance (Stackhouse, 1998). Until the passage of the Balanced Budget Act (BBA) of 1997, home care was the fastest growing segment of the healthcare industry, with the number of Medicare-certified home health agencies increasing from 1,753 in 1967 to 10,000 in 1997. According to the National Association for Home Care (2002) by the year 2000, the number had dropped back to approximately 7,000 agencies. The BBA instituted the Prospective Payment System for Medicare-covered home care, with the impact on reimbursement being swift and deep. Eighty Home Health Resource Groups were developed based on data from the Outcome and Assessment Information Set (OASIS). The Balanced Budget Refinement Act (BBRA) of 1999 brought some relief to home health agencies, restoring an estimated 1.3 billion in Medicare payment reductions (Giacalone, 2001).

CHARACTERISTICS OF PATIENTS

To qualify for Medicare reimbursed home services, the recipient of care must require skilled nursing care, physical therapy, or speech therapy. Examples of skilled nursing care include: creation of a plan of care, assessment and monitoring, medication administration, infusion therapy, teaching, wound care, ventilator care, tracheostomy care, supporting bowel and bladder function including foley catheter care, tube feedings, chest physiotherapy and inhalation therapy, and diabetic management. Additional specialized long-term patient needs may involve hospice care for terminally ill patients and psychiatric/mental health services. The recipient of care must be confined to home and have a physician's order for home health care (Stackhouse, 1998). Common conditions requiring longer-term management in the home include stroke, diabetes, heart disease, and mental and cognitive disorders.

Elders receiving home-care services in the U.S. doubled from two million in 1990 to four million in 1997. Since the passage of the Balanced Budget Act in 1997, the numbers have begun to decline (Giacalone, 2001).

NURSE STAFFING

Registered nurses in home care prepare and coordinate a multidisciplinary plan of care. Home health aides provide personal care, e.g., assistance with bathing and grooming, meal preparation, some basic housekeeping and other tasks as delegated by the home health nurse. In 1998, there were 518,640 home health agency caregivers: 62.9 percent were NAs, 24.9 percent were RNs, 7.9 percent were LPNs, and 4.2 percent were physical therapists or social workers (Wunderlich & Kohler, 2001). The Bureau of Labor Statistics expects the demand for RNs in home health services to increase by 82 percent between 1998 and 2008. Currently, more than 68 percent of home health agencies are reporting problems in recruiting and retaining home health aides (Kovner & Harrington, 2002).

QUALITY OF CARE

The use of the Outcomes Assessment Information Set (OASIS) is mandated for Medicare certification. Just as in other settings, quality management involves assuring competent staff, auditing procedures, risk management, and utilization review. A new assessment instrument, the Minimum Data Set for Home Care (MDS-HC), patterned after the MDS used in nursing homes is currently being implemented (Landi et al., 2001).

A study by Morrow-Howell, Proctor, and Rozario (2001) compared ratings of sufficiency of home care between nursing professionals and elderly recipients of care. Elderly patients rated the sufficiency of care higher than the nurses. Elkan and colleagues (2001) found that home visits to frail elders reduced mortality and admissions to institutional care. On the other hand, a 2001 study of severely disabled stroke patients by Chiu, Shyu, and Liu suggested that home care is less appropriate and cost-effective than institutional care for people with severe disabilities.

ASSISTED LIVING

Another arrangement for delivering long-term care services is the combination of care and housing, in a congregate, but less restrictive setting than a nursing home, i.e., assisted living or adult care homes. An assisted living setting combines a homelike environment and the capacity for health-care services, while offering private living space and greater control and choice (Kane, Kane, & Ladd, 1998; Allen, 1999). The Assisted Living Federation of America defines this brand of long-term care as the combination of housing, personalized support services, and health care designed to meet the individual needs of residents who need help with activities of daily living, but who do not need skilled nursing care. The concept of "aging in place" is a cornerstone of assisted living (Chen & Cohen, 2002). In the U.S., the approximately 5,000 assisted living facilities, licensed and monitored by state and local governments, provide assistance with activities of daily living and medication administration, but do not provide the skilled and comprehensive health care of a nursing home (North Carolina Assisted Living News, 2002). State regulations focus on three main areas: living unit requirements, resident admission and retention criteria, and the types and levels of services provided (U.S. General Accounting Office, 1997).

There are approximately another 20,000 provider types that are known as residential care facilities, congregate living facilities, rest homes, personal care homes, board and care homes, and domiciliary care (Long Term Care Education.com, 2002). Adult day care, with roots in Great Britain's geriatric day hospital concept, is another element now on the scene of the long-term care continuum in the United States. According to the National Institute of Adult Day Care, this level of care is another form of long term care offered for periods less than 24 hours. Assisted living facilities, as an important component of the continuum of care and an alternative to inappropriate or premature nursing home placement, were introduced into the United States in the 1980s, based on a Scandinavian model of long-term care (Giacalone, 2001).

According to assisted living data cited by Kovner and Harrington (2003), close to a million older adults lived in one of approximately 33,000 assisted living facilities in the U.S. in 2001. Women, at an average age of 84, account for 78 percent of the residents of assisted living facilities. Male residents are slightly younger, on average. The typical assisted living resident profile is someone who needs assistance with three activities of daily living and takes six daily medications.

Kingston, Bernard, Biggs, and Nettleton (2001) found that older people living in assisted living facilities compared favorably with community dwelling elders in terms of maintaining physical and mental health. Autonomy combined with peer support and safety and security were identified as key factors in maintaining health status.

SUMMARY

The researcher seeking to gain entry into the world of a nursing home in order to conduct research will be well-served by developing an understanding and appreciation of the nursing home environment. Such an understanding should include some knowledge of the regulatory process and its strong influence on the corporate culture of the nursing home. The researcher should appreciate resource constraints and the fact that nursing home work is hard work, and thus staff turnover is often much higher than in other segments of health care. Nursing home residents are typically frail and often cognitively impaired. Nursing home personnel who achieve longevity in the long-term care setting typically possess a special brand of dedication and can be extremely useful resource people. A researcher with an interest in long-term care settings should be prepared for the impact of the heavy care needs of chronically ill residents and the influence of a high prevalence of dementia. Similar phenomena exist in community-based long-term care settings, but typically to a lesser degree.

Chapter 2

The State of the Science of Long-Term Care Research

Compared with other health care settings, long-term care settings have been underutilized for research, especially controlled clinical studies. However, nursing homes in particular can be rich sources of clinical data, mostly due to longstanding regulatory requirements to track information about residents and their care. According to McBride (2000), the gerontological research agenda in general should focus on preventing disease and disability where possible, as well as minimizing morbidity and maximizing quality of life in the presence of disabling conditions. The message was clear among participants in a Spring 2002 workshop sponsored by the Clinical Research Roundtable of the Institute of Medicine: researchers must put more emphasis on improvements in the treatment of chronic conditions in the elderly (Eastman, 2002).

Long-term care researchers should be forerunners in the generation, testing, and dissemination of knowledge in the field of gerontology. Long-term care settings provide rich and varied milieus and patient populations. This chapter will introduce the reader to thematic areas of research being conducted in long-term care settings. It will provide a review of the patterns and trends of recent research studies conducted primarily in nursing homes, but will also reference studies conducted in home care and assisted living.

RESEARCH PRIORITIES IN LONG-TERM CARE

Phillips and Van Ort (1995) discussed the nursing home as a nearly perfect research laboratory for the study of clinical management of chronic conditions, since it is characterized by long-staying residents in a self-contained, circumscribed, potentially controllable environment. Such an environment presents many problems amenable to intervention and the opportunity to test the results of interventions over time. Nursing homes offer advantages not possible in settings with more rapid turnover of patients (such as hospitals) or with many more uncontrollable external influences (such as the home). Long-term care research includes descriptive studies aimed at a better understanding of problems experienced by chronically ill patients as well as clinical trials directed toward improved treatment of chronic conditions. The state of the science of clinical research in long-term care is addressed in this chapter.

In addition, long-term care research encompasses health services research aimed at assessing the organization and delivery of care in terms of quality and outcomes. Trends in health services research are also highlighted in this chapter.

CLINICAL STUDIES IN LONG-TERM CARE

Clinical research addresses patients' health problems and responses to treatment. Regardless of the setting in which care is provided, recipients of long-term care exhibit common, chronic health problems. There have been a variety of clinical studies regarding these common problems; however, many of the studies have been descriptive in nature or have involved small samples of mostly nursing home residents. Common health conditions observed in long-term care are listed in Table 2.1, providing the long-term care researcher with an overview of recurring clinical problems as a focus of research and providing a framework for the discussion of clinical research in long-term care. According to Ignaviticius (1998), common health problems include falls, pressure ulcers, urinary incontinence, cognitive impairment, malnutrition, and loss of normal bowel function. Other challenges include infection control and pain management. The studies cited in this chapter are not an exhaustive set of references, but rather highlight examples of studies and findings related to each topic.

Decreased Mobility, Falls, and Restraints

Declining mobility is a major clinical issue in long-term care, resulting in self-care limitations and diminution of quality of life for patients or residents, and heavier care demands for staff. Typically, functional ability is measured through activities of daily living (such as hygiene and personal

TABLE 2.1   Common Health Problems of Frail Elders

Acute/minor emergency
  Falls
  Fever
  Musculoskeletal pain

Circulation
  Chest pain
  Hypertension
  Hypotension
  Edema (new onset)

Elimination
  Incontinence
  Constipation
  Diarrhea

Nutrition
  Dehydration
  Hyperglycemia
  Hypoglycemia
  Unexpected weight loss

Psychosocial
  Depressed mood/reactive depression
  Combative/aggressive behavior
  Delirium, acute altered mental status
  Insomnia (acute disturbance of sleep pattern)

Respiratory
  Nasal/sinus congestion
  Shortness of breath

Sensory/Integumentary
  Dry, itchy eyes
  Localized rash (perineal or under breasts)
  Skin tears
  Pressure ulcers

care) as well as instrumental activities of daily living (those activities necessary to manage in the community such as shopping, personal finances, and meal preparation). It is reasonable to assume that basic activities of daily living constitute a more relevant measurement in a nursing home facility; instrumental activities of daily living remain more relevant in more independent settings such as the home and assisted living centers. A study published in 2000 by Magaziner and colleagues showed that the vast majority of nursing home residents require assistance with basic activities of daily living: 96 percent with bathing, 87 percent with dressing, 74 percent with transferring, 63 percent with toileting, and 46 percent with eating. Schwarz (2000) explored hospital readmissions of functionally impaired older adults ($n = 71$), the majority of whom were receiving home care services. Schwarz found a significant inverse relationship between increased tangible support, such as transportation services and hospitalization.

Mobility and the ability to carry out activities of daily living (functional status) are measured through instruments such as the Katz Index of Activities of Daily Living (Katz, Ford, Moskowitz, Jackson, & Jaffe, 1963). Impaired mobility, combined with multiple medications and, in many cases, alterations in judgment associated with dementia, results in a negative spiral of greater numbers of falls and more restrictive interventions. Cohen, Gorenberg, and Schroeder (2000) examined the quality of life related to functional status among community-dwelling elders ($n = 68$) who were clients of nurse-managed centers in California. Using the Older American Resources and Services (OARS) tool, an instrument developed with support from multiple federal agencies, the nurse researchers confirmed the relationship between functional ability and quality of life. Using comprehensive assessments, such as OARS, for planning and coordination of care can enhance functional status and quality of life. In a much larger scale study published in 2002, Mathieson, Kronenfeld, and Keith investigated the roles of health status and financial resources on functional independence in a nationally representative sample ($n = 3,485$) of non-institutionalized adults age 65 and over. Effective promotion of functional adaptations evolves from early targeting of elders with few limitations as well as consideration of financial factors in addition to health status. Assisted living arrangements were shown to benefit low income elders' maintenance of functional ability or management of functional decline in a study by Fonda, Clipp, and Maddox (2002).

Although federal regulatory reform issued a clear message about the undesirability of physical and/or chemical restraints, and since virtually nobody believes that mechanisms to restrict movement are humane, the prevention of falls and related injuries is a complex challenge in long-term care. In nursing homes in particular, part of the dilemma stems from families' unrealistic expectations that a resident will never fall and fears of litigation by the nursing home staff.

Falls are an important concern, often resulting in physical injuries such as head trauma, fractures, and soft tissue damage, as well as psychological trauma related to fear of falling. Fall-related injuries are the leading cause of injury, deaths, and disabilities among people over 65 (Stevens & Olson, 2000). Falls may result from musculoskeletal or neurological changes that affect balance and coordination, reaction time, sensory abilities, or judgment. Related factors include infections, incontinence, pain, and the use of drugs that cause hypotension or sedation. Environmental hazards such as glare, slippery surfaces, lack of supervision and assistive devices, and even inappropriate footwear contribute to fall risk (Tinetti, Doucette, & Claus, 1995). Frail elders are particularly vulnerable to falls and to serious injuries from falls, especially hip fractures, which are related not only to advancing age, but also to low body mass index, a history of osteoporosis, and a previous hip fracture. Caucasian women over 65 are the highest risk group.

Primary prevention of falls includes increasing physical activity to improve strength, balance, and coordination; environmental modification; education regarding fall prevention; and reduction of specific risk factors. Secondary prevention involves reducing fall-related injuries and includes padding and hip protectors and even innovations such as special energy-absorbing flooring (Stevens & Olson, 2000).

Ray and colleagues (1997) conducted a randomized trial of a consultation service to reduce falls in nursing homes. They selected seven pairs of nursing homes in Tennessee for the study, and randomly assigned one facility in each pair to the intervention. There were 221 subjects in the experimental group and 261 controls. Residents in both groups qualified for the study because of a high risk for falling, a risk that could potentially be reduced by the intervention. The intervention consisted of comprehensive individual assessment followed by specific environmental and personal safety recommendations. Targeted practices included the use of psychotropic drugs, the use of a wheelchair, transferring, and ambulation. The mean proportion of recurrent fallers in the nursing homes receiving the intervention was over 19 percent lower than that of control facilities, revealing the effectiveness of intervention research in nursing homes.

A 1999 study by Resnick described the incidence of falls in a sample of 220 older adults living in an assisted living environment in a continuing care retirement community. Over a two-year period, 154 falls were documented using a falls data form. Most of the falls took place in the residents' apartments between noon and midnight. The majority (63 percent) of the falls occurred while the resident was walking; 19 percent occurred during the act of transferring. Only 10 percent of the falls resulted in fractures, but there was a significant relationship between repeated falling and suffering an injurious fall. Multiple falls were associated with neurological problems, heart arrhythmias, being unmarried, and not adhering to a regular exercise program. The findings offer insight in terms of determining fall risk and designing interventions appropriate for assisted living facilities as well as home care settings.

Nursing home residents with a history of mobility problems and falls as well as cognitive impairment and use of psychotropic medications are significantly more likely to be physically restrained, even after OBRA nursing home reform (Castle, Fogel, & Mor, 1997). Restraint-free nursing homes typically have higher-functioning residents, are smaller in size, have nonprofit status, have lower occupancy, are located in an urban setting, and have more registered nurses in the staff mix (Castle & Fogel, 1998).

A 1996 descriptive correlational study by Phillips and colleagues addressed the relationship between characteristics and geographic location of nursing home facilities and the use of physical restraints. After controlling for residents' physical and cognitive function, the researchers found that restraint practices varied widely by geographical area, and that facilities with low nurse staffing were more likely to restrain residents. In a study of the use of restraints in the preceding year, Graber and Sloane (1995) found that the ratio of nursing staff to residents and the overall disability level in the facility were factors associated with overall use of restraints. Other factors associated with regulatory deficiencies for the use of physical restraints were the size of the facility, the cost per patient/day, the proportion of restrained residents, the proportion of residents with dementia, and the use of bladder training in less than three percent of the residents. Factors of borderline significance were profit status, the proportion of residents who were intubated, and the proportion of residents on psychotropic medication. Nursing researchers in Finland used a qualitative approach to examine nursing home staff ($n = 20$) perceptions of the use of restraints. Their findings indicated a need for greater attention to the rights and responsibilities of both residents and staff (Hantikainen & Kappeli, 2000).

Dunbar, Neufeld, White, and Libow (1996) were able to achieve a 90 percent reduction in the use of restraints through an educational intervention applied in sixteen randomly selected nursing homes in a national demonstration study over a two-year period. The intervention involved a workshop, telephone as well as quarterly on-site consultations, regional meetings, a newsletter, and written and audiovisual materials that advocated interdisciplinary assessments to generate individually tailored restraint-free interventions. A number of similar research and demonstration projects employing multiple strategies with positive results have recently been supported by the Centers for Medicare and Medicaid.

A study of chemical restraints in nursing homes, conducted in 2000 by the Office of the Inspector General of the U.S. Department of Health and Human Services, concluded that 85 percent of psychotropic drug use is appropriate. However, the National Citizens Coalition for Nursing Home Reform, reacted that the report failed to identify the important relationship between staffing ratios and the ability to reduce the number of chemical restraints. A 1997 study of 2,054 residents in a total of 410 other long-term care facilities (board and care) in 10 states, found inappropriate drug regimens, often involving psychotropic medications in between 20–25 percent of residents. Medication use in general may create a slippery slope for frail elders. Polypharmacy or use of multiple medications and often inappropriate use of drugs or combinations of drugs are problems especially among older people. Nearly one third of 6,718 elderly home health-care patients, surveyed in 2001 by Meredith and colleagues, were taking a drug that was inappropriate for geriatric populations or had some other medication problem. The subjects in the study took a median of five medications, while an astounding 19 percent of them took nine or more medications.

Other Hazards of Immobility

Intact skin is the body's first line of defense against physiological threats such as infection and underlying tissue damage. With increasing age, there is a decrease in subcutaneous tissue and skin is simply more fragile, as evidenced for example, by the number and frequency of tears in the skin. Interruptions in skin integrity, including pressure ulcers related to decreased mobility, are common in chronically ill people. Malnutrition and a negative nitrogen balance and shearing force/friction to the skin are also important epidemiological factors in the development of pressure ulcers. Pressure ulcers increase pain and vulnerability in frail elders in nursing homes as well as at home and in hospitals, result in soaring costs of care, and are frequently cited in litigation against the health-care industry. Therefore, beyond the obvious benefits, the prevention of pressure ulcers has been shown to significantly reduce health care costs (Xakellis, Frantz, Lewis, & Harvey, 1998).

The Braden Scale for Predicting Pressure Ulcer Risk (Bergstrom, Braden, Laguzza, & Holman, 1987) is a widely used instrument and an instrument with which a clinical researcher in long-term care should be familiar. Using the Braden pressure ulcer scale, investigators have been able to identify residents at risk for pressure ulcer formation so that risk-reduction measures could be implemented to reduce the incidence and prevalence of pressure ulcers (Kartes, 1996). This practice is supported in recommendations of the National Pressure Ulcer Advisory Panel. However, in a study of 555 nursing home residents, Vap and Dunaye (2000) did not find additive value in the Braden Scale over data collected in the Minimum Data Set; however the MDS tended to overpredict residents at risk for pressure ulcer development.

A multisite study of the predictive validity of the Braden Scale was published by Bergstom and Braden in 2002. A total of 843 Caucasian and African-American subjects in nursing homes, tertiary care centers, and Veterans Administration Medical Centers in Omaha, Chicago, and Raleigh were studied. A score of 18 on the Braden scale identified individuals at risk for pressure ulcers, although white subjects had a higher actual incidence of pressure ulcers.

Incontinence

Independence with toileting is characteristic of a minority of nursing home residents and many community-dwelling older adults, especially women. According to Medical Expenditure Panel Survey findings, more than half of nursing home residents experience bladder and/or bowel incontinence. Unfortunately, lack of bladder and/or bowel control may be perceived as an inevitable consequence of aging and not as a treatable or manageable condition. Although urinary incontinence, the involuntary loss of urine, is not a normal physiological change associated with aging, it is common among community dwelling elders, especially women.

Direct observations in a 1999 study by Simmons and Schnelle revealed low frequencies in care related to maintaining both mobility and continence. Resnick (2001) cited the need for greater emphasis on restorative care, which, in contrast to fostering learned helplessness and dependence, seeks to reestablish and maintain function, while compensating for impaired function. Mueller and Cam (2002) identified quality improvement factors related to urinary incontinence in long-term care facilities: evidence-based practice, assessment, environmental interventions, education, staffing, communication, involvement, and evaluation/feedback.

Incontinence was the subject of a 1995 clinical study by Ouslander and colleagues, who developed a simple noninvasive assessment technique that allowed nursing home staff members to identify 191 incontinent residents from seven nursing homes who would be likely to respond to prompted voiding. The results revealed that 41 percent of the residents responded to a prompted voiding protocol. The wetness proportion among residents dropped from 26.7 percent to 6.4 percent at the end of one week and was maintained at 9.6 percent following nine weeks of prompted voiding. The best predictors of responsiveness to prompted voiding were the pre-study wet percentages, the appropriate toileting behavior percentage during the first three days of the intervention, independent ambulation, and self-care. Prompted voiding is typically used only during daytime hours and even with this intervention, incontinence often remains a problem during the night. In 1998, Schnelle, Cruise, Alessi, Al-Samarrai, and Ouslander investigated strategies for reducing sleep disruption related to incontinence care among 92 residents in four nursing home facilities. Awakenings for incontinence care were significantly reduced without adverse effects on healthy skin.

In 2000, Lyons and Pringle-Specht refined a research-based protocol for prompted voiding which begins with a thorough assessment, including patterns of incontinent episodes, followed by the implementation of a behavioral intervention in which typically incontinent individuals are prompted to void prior to involuntary loss of urine, and finally by evaluation of the reduction in the frequency and volume of incontinence. Positive social feedback and staff management are important components in the success of a prompted voiding protocol. This protocol is adaptable for use in long-term care settings.

In a 2001 study, Jerovic and Templin evaluated the effects of a similar toileting program, individualized scheduled voiding, among 108 incontinent, memory-impaired elders receiving home health care. Moderately impaired elders, able to cooperate with toileting protocols were determined to most likely benefit from such a program.

A clinical practice guideline on urinary incontinence was released by the then Agency for Health Care Policy Research in 1996. The application of the guideline was evaluated in 52 nursing homes in a study by Watson, published in 2002. Overall, 31 percent of the most important guideline standards were met. Major barriers to implementation were lack of knowledge and insufficient resources.

Cognitive Impairment/Mental Disorders

Cognitive impairment is a major issue in long-term care. Dementia from Alzheimer's disease and other related disorders is, by a variety of estimates, present in well over half of nursing home residents; the prevalence of depression is high as well (Magaziner et al., 2000). Dementia manifests itself in memory loss, disorientation, problems with language and communication, decreasing functional ability, impaired judgment, and behavior and mood changes. The course of Alzheimer's disease, with its characteristic amyloid plaques and neurofibrillary tangles that form in the brain, involves three broad stages ranging from short-term memory loss in the early stage, to more profound memory impairment, language difficulties, and behavioral changes in the middle stage, to the loss of mobility and complete care requirements in the late or terminal stage. Medical Expenditure Panel Survey data, involving nationally representative assessments of medical care use and expenditures (described in Chapter 1), reveal that cognitive problems are more prevalent than actual behavior problems among nursing home residents. The Mini Mental Status Examination (Folstein, Folstein, & McHugh, 1975) is the instrument most commonly used to measure cognitive impairment. It contains 22 questions administered by a clinician that assess thinking and memory.

A descriptive study by Kovach and Krejci in 1998 explored factors that facilitate improvements or positive changes in dementia care, according to 181 long-term care employees. Findings supported the tenets of strong leadership, communication, involvement, and empowerment as the foundations of effective care. Another 1998 study by Anderson, Wendler, and Congdon suggested that there is a gap between research and actual practice, following observations of the responses of nursing home staff to the behaviors of agitation, aggression, screaming, wandering, and repetitive actions of residents with Alzheimer's Disease. Such behaviors, typically perceived as creating challenges for staff, may also contribute to the overall decline of the resident as they may lead to exhaustion, social isolation, and physical harm.

Voelkl, Galecki, and Fries (1996) found that, in a sample of 3,008 nursing home residents, those with severe cognitive impairment spent significantly less time in organized activities. To better understand the predictors of participation in activity, they went on to study a subsample of 1,210 cognitively impaired nursing home residents. Predictors included utilization group category, location preferences, sense of involvement, and the type of nursing home unit. The database for this study came from the Health Care Financing Administration's Multi-State Nursing Home Case-Mix and Quality Demonstration Project.

While there are increasing clinical practice guidelines for dementia care, the development of such guidelines is only a first step toward implementation. In a survey of 200 facilities in the Veterans Administration, Rosen and colleagues .(2002) determined that the majority of the VA centers routinely conducted neurological examinations, including cognitive screening and screening for depression, obtained histories from caregivers, discussed the diagnosis and treatment with the family, and addressed legal and decision-making issues. Prescribing of medications was also broadly consistent with recommended guidelines. However, caregiver support was included in the plan of care only 50 percent of the time. Patient and family education and support and coaching of caregivers is as much a part of practice guidelines, especially in regard to dementia, as assessment and treatment.

Mental health and communication problems are common among nursing home residents and plague other chronically ill older adults as well. Social relatedness is an important concept to gerontologists and nursing home researchers. The Geriatric Rating Scale (Plutchik et al., 1970) is a 12-item rating scale, based on staff observation, often used to measure social engagement.

A 1995 study of social engagement among nursing home residents sought to test the reliability and construct validity of social engagement, a measure of the quality of life which can be isolated from the Resident Assessment Instrument. Using a sample of 1,848 residents from 268 nursing homes in ten states, the researchers hypothesized a four-factor model with social engagement distinguished from mood problems, conflicted relationships, and behavior problems. For high-functioning residents, social engagement was negatively related to conflict, but the two were positive related among the most impaired (Mor et al., 1995). A study reported in 1997 by Resnick, Fries, and Verbrugge examined hearing, visual, and communication abilities, social engagement, and time spent in activities. The combined effects of visual and communication impairments were associated with low social engagement. Vision impairment was also found by Horowitz (1997) to be associated with disruptive behaviors.

In 2001, Biliipp studied the effect of an innovation in which home health nurses taught their vulnerable elderly clients computer skills after installation of telecommunication terminals in clients' homes. The interactive computer increased communication opportunities for social as well as functional or health-care-related purposes. The result was a significant improvement in self-esteem and depression.

Signs and symptoms of depression include a flat affect, loss of energy, a pervasive sense of hopelessness, and appetite and sleep disturbances. Depression is often evaluated with the Geriatric Depression Scale (Yesavage & Brink, 1983). In the short form, the instrument contains 15 yes/no items. The Philadelphia Geriatric Center Morale Scale (Lawton, 1975) contains 23 yes/no items. The latter two instruments, like other instruments of these formats, require the ability to understand the meaning of the questions. Much of the present work in instrument development for geriatric populations is focused on tools suitable for subjects with significant cognitive impairment.

Dehydration and Weight Loss

Optimal nutrition and hydration among nursing home residents constitute major clinical challenges, with the prevalence of malnutrition up to 50 percent reported in the literature owing to the pervasiveness of chronic conditions, including depression. Weinberg and Minaker (1996) conducted an integrated review of the literature regarding dehydration. They concluded that dehydration may go unrecognized because physical signs are often absent or misleading among older patients. When residents are identified as being at risk for possible dehydration, an interdisciplinary care plan is critical. Also in 1996, Roubenoff, Giacoppe, Richardson, and Hoffman addressed the challenging problem of nutrition assessment in long-term care facilities with new techniques of measuring macronutrient status, such as indirect calorimetry. Roubenoff and colleagues framed their work within the emerging focus in health care on cost effectiveness and the need to demonstrate that improved nutrition assessment is related to better nutritional outcomes.

McCann, Hawes, and Groth-Juncker, in a 1994 study of 32 terminally ill patients, found that the majority did not experience hunger or thirst; among those who did, small amounts of food, sips of liquid, and mouth care promoted comfort. In a related study, professional caregivers in thirteen nursing homes in Stockholm, Sweden, were asked to evaluate a situation in which a resident of sound mind refused to eat or drink. While 50 percent of the respondents believed that the resident's decision should be respected, only 20 percent projected that, in actuality, there would be no intervention on the part of the caregivers (Mattiasson & Andersson, 1994).

A 1995, large-scale secondary analysis of MDS data from 6,832 nursing home residents in 202 nursing homes in seven states revealed that poor oral intake, chewing problems, dependency in eating, and pressure ulcers were related to weight loss and low body mass index. Low body mass index was associated with female gender, advancing age (85 or older), hip fracture, and bedridden status, whereas depression and two or more chronic diseases increased the odds of weight loss. The researchers, Blaum, Fries, and Fiatarone (1995), concluded that undernutrition is a multifactorial phenomenon among nursing home residents and recommended improved oral feeding methods and the treatment of depression.

The decision factors in using a feeding tube to combat dehydration and undernutrition in nursing home residents with severe cognitive impairment were studied by Gessert, Mosier, Brown, and Frey (2000) and Ahronheim, Mulvihill, Sieger, Park, and Fries (2001). Gessert and colleagues tracked 4,997 residents of Kansas nursing homes who suffered from severe cognitive impairment, 577 (11.6 percent) of whom had feeding tubes. Based on data collected from the Minimum Data Set, feeding tube use was associated with swallowing problems (stroke), urban location of nursing homes, non-White race, milder dementia, and, to a lesser degree, with age greater than 86 years, male gender, total dependence in activities of daily living, and the absence of a living will. Ahronheim and colleagues investigated the prevalence of tube feeding in nine states, encompassing a total of 57,029 residents. The prevalence ranged from 7.5 percent in Maine to 40.1 percent in Mississippi, revealing wide regional variations in the practice.

Infectious Diseases

Infectious diseases, particularly those caused by drug-resistant organisms, are becoming a crisis in nursing home facilities where residents are elderly and typically have multiple comorbidities. Nicolle, Bentley, Garibaldi, Neuhaus, and Smith (1996) noted that attempts to improve the use of antimicrobials in nursing homes are complicated by characteristics of the resident population, the limited availability of diagnostic tests, and the virtual absence of relevant clinical trials. The authors recommended approaches to the management of common infections in nursing homes and proposed minimum standards for an antimicrobial review program. Li, Birkhead, Strogatz, and Coles (1996) found that facility size, staffing patterns, and employee sick leave policies were the principal risk factors for the occurrence of nosocomial respiratory or gastrointestinal disease. Loeb and colleagues (2001) identified colonization with multiresistant bacteria as a quality of life issue for nursing home residents. Stevenson (1999) described the development of a regional data set of infection rates for long-term care facilities as important benchmarking information. Stevenson's work illustrates an interface of research addressing common clinical problems with a health services approach.

Pain

Pain is an understudied phenomenon in nursing homes. However, depressive symptoms and pain are the most common resident complaints, even though pain may actually be under-reported by elders. Loeb (1999) described the phenomena of pain among nursing home residents being underdetected and undertreated as well. Stein and Ferrell (1996) offered an integrated review of studies regarding the treatment of pain in the nursing home setting. They postulated that pharmacological treatments for pain are limited, owing to the higher incidence of side effects with elderly persons. A more recent study (Cook, 1998) found that nursing home residents without serious cognitive impairment respond well to cognitive and behavioral pain-management strategies.

The aim of a large-scale study by Fries, Simon, Morris, Flodstrom, and Bookstein (2001) involved validation of a pain scale for use with the Minimum Data Set in nursing home populations. A visual analogue pain scale based on data derived from 95 nursing home residents with intact communication skills was then used in a retrospective analysis of 34,675 Michigan nursing home residents. The implications of the Fries study suggest that pain is prevalent in nursing home residents, but often untreated, especially in cognitively impaired residents. According to Ross and Crook (1998), pain among elders receiving home health services is also under-recognized. Three quarters of the 66 individuals interviewed in their study reported that pain was linked to decreased functional ability and quality of life, as well as feelings of depression and sleep disturbances.

HEALTH SERVICES RESEARCH

Health services research is concerned with broad, population-based outcomes of care delivery, and seeks to improve health-care delivery and to evaluate the impact of health policy (Curry, 2002). It focuses on the organization and financing of health services, health-care access and quality, informatics and clinical decision-making, clinical evaluation and outcomes, provider/practitioner and consumer behavior, the health professions workforce, health policy formulation and analysis, health-care modeling, and use of services (Cody, Beck, Courtney, & Shue, 2002). The nursing home environment and other settings in which long-term care is delivered as part of the continuum of health care lend themselves to health services research as well as clinical research. Rather than focusing on specific clinical problems and related interventions, health services research focuses on how health care, in this case, long-term care, is organized and delivered. Binstock and Spector (1997) recommended five priority areas for health services research in long-term care: the development and refinement of quality-of-care measures, cost and demand, cost and quality of care across settings, innovations in care, and managed care in long-term care settings. In 1997 the Agency for Health Care Policy and Research, later renamed the Agency for Healthcare Research and Quality, identified long-term care research priorities that were similar, but included questions about access, the organization of care delivery, consumer and caregiver behavior, and special populations. The agency emphasized methodological and data-development issues. For example, Schnelle and colleagues (1999) compared the quality of care of nursing home residents enrolled in managed care plans with traditional fee-for-service arrangements, finding that while the former group fared better on most objective measures of quality, consumer perceptions did not detect the difference. Castle, Mor, and Banaszak-Holl (1997) provided a descriptive analysis of nursing homes that contained special care hospice units. Being small in size, proprietary, part of a chain, and located in a more competitive environment were all significant factors relating to having a hospice special care unit. Alzheimer's special care units have also been studied by several researchers (Grant, Kane, & Stark, 1995; Mehr & Fries, 1995; Sloane, Lindeman, Phillips, Moritz, & Koch, 1995).

In 1999, Friedermann, Montgomery, Rice, and Farrell, studied family involvement in the delivery of long-term care to nursing home residents. Based on a conceptual model that applied systems theory, interviews were conducted with 216 family members of residents in 24 Michigan nursing homes. Pre-established family behavior and dynamics were the best predictors of the family's expected involvement in care. Expected involvement, combined with the family caregiver relationship and the functional ability of the resident, accounted for most of the variance in actual family involvement in the delivery of care. When hospice care is integrated into nursing home care, hospitalizations decrease for Medicare patients, according to a 2001 study by Miller, Gozalo, and Mor, comparing 9,202 hospice residents with 27,500 nonhospice residents in five states. Teno (2002) challenged that it is time to embrace nursing homes as a place of care for dying persons.

Telemedicine, the use of distance technologies such as interactive video, has been the focus of health services research in home care. Results of a study conducted in the Veteran's Administration by Noel and Vogel (2000) suggest that integrating telemedicine with nurse case management can decrease the costs of care and reduce hospitalizations among elderly homebound patients. The TeleHomecare Project (Hale, Fong, & Dansky, 2001), a partnership among Penn State University, American Telecare, and the Visiting Nurses Association, evaluated the use of telecommunications as a supplement to skilled nursing visits for home-care patients with diabetes. The experimental variable of telecommunications was compared with customary care in a total of 171 diabetic patients. Patients who used the telecommunications technology demonstrated better control of diabetes, fewer visits to emergency rooms, and fewer hospitalizations.

Measurement of Quality and Outcomes of Long-Term Care

In long-term care settings, as along the rest of the health-care continuum, research efforts are increasingly focused on evidence-based care or outcomes research (Castle, Zinn, Brannon, & Mor, 1997). Harrington and colleagues (1999) found that stakeholders representing diverse and sometimes adversarial positions agreed on the three most important measures of how well the nation's nursing homes are doing their jobs. Nursing home administrators, nursing service directors, regulators, ombudsmen (i.e., advocacy positions created by the Older Americans Act) (Lieberman, 2000), and other advocates alike ranked quality of care provided by staff, quality of life of residents, and residents' rights as the three most important quality concepts. However, measuring outcomes of nursing home care is challenging in that outcome indicators that have been developed for other arenas may not apply to a high-risk population in which dementia and frailty are increasingly prevalent. In long-term care, the researcher is faced with trying to determine objective measures of the quality of care that are interwoven with subjective measures of the quality of life so important in this population.

Nursing homes, in part due to heavy regulation, have abundant structure and process measures but research has been slow in using these data to augment traditional outcome measures such as mortality and hospital admissions. Since quality of life is such an important variable, satisfaction surveys are a particularly relevant measure among nursing home residents, families, and significant others. However, satisfaction surveys are often inadequate not only because of the high prevalence of dementia, but also a generally low response rate and a lack of specificity of measurement instruments. There may be some acquiescence or perceived threat among respondents.

In 2001, the Institute of Medicine suggested three aspects of long-term care relevant to assessing quality: (1) long-term care involves both health and social programs; therefore measures of quality include both health and functional outcomes as well as satisfaction and quality of life; (2) the potential and actual roles of consumers are essential elements in long-term care; and (3) for nursing homes and other residential care facilities, the physical environment plays a role in quality as it contributes to the mobility and physical safety of residents as well as to their quality of life (e.g., privacy). Quality improvement guidelines for nursing homes, ranging from assessment to quality of care to staffing, were essential components of OBRA '87 (Jaffe, 1998). The MDS, a central feature of OBRA and one of the most sweeping changes of the law, is designed to improve outcomes of nursing home care through standardized indicators of clinical care quality (Rantz & Popejoy, 1998).

Miller, Coe, Morley, and Romeis (1995) proposed the following model for developing initiatives to improve quality in the nursing home setting:

1. Select the topic
2. Organize the team
3. Develop standards with staff input
4. Distribute standards
5. Collect data
6. Analyze and summarize data
7. Identify problems
8. Give feedback to staff
9. Plan and implement
10. Implement corrective strategies
11. Collect further data
12. Re-evaluate

Writing on the development and testing of nursing home quality indicators, Zimmerman and colleagues (1995) described the evolution of quality indicators as the result of two related developments in relation to nursing home quality. The first development is a growing interest among health care professionals, consumers, policy makers, and other advocates in issues related to the quality of care and the quality of life of nursing home residents. The second development is the implementation of a case-mix classification system to serve as a basis for Medicare and Medicaid payments as well as a quality measurement system to assess the impact of case-mix on quality, as evidenced by the Multi-State Nursing Home Case Mix and Quality Demonstration funded by the Health Care Financing Administration (HCFA). Initially six states participated in the demonstration project.

The key elements of the quality-measurement system are the quality indicators, and these are derived from items on the Minimum Data Set (MDS) described in Chapter 1. Since the MDS has evolved through several iterations, it has been redesigned to be more than an individual assessment instrument. In its current form, it is also a measure of the use of resources and includes important indicators of the quality of care. A total of 175 quality indicators are organized within the following twelve care domains:

1. Accidents
2. Behavioral and Emotional Patterns
3. Clinical Management
4. Cognitive Functioning
5. Elimination and Continence
6. Infection Control
7. Nutrition and Eating
8. Physical Functioning
9. Psychotropic Drug Use
10. Quality of Life
11. Sensory Function and Communication
12. Skin Care

Being able to determine the quality of care from routine assessment information collected among nursing home residents has the potential to play a vital role in improving resident outcomes and to dramatically influence public policy decisions regarding reimbursement, recertification, and regulation. The American Health Care Association Quality Indicator Index in Education project showed that the limited intervention of introducing quantitative care measurements and tracking quality indicator information from the MDS had a significant impact on resident outcomes and the nursing process when tested in nine nursing facilities in Mississippi (Fitzgerald, Shiverick, & Zimmerman, 1996; Karon & Zimmerman, 1998). Rantz and colleagues (1996) described the assessment of the quality of nursing home care as the foundation for improving resident outcomes in a study that analyzed quality indicators identified by the HCFA-sponsored Case Mix and Quality Demonstration Project. Using the Missouri Nursing Home Minimum Database, Rantz and colleagues found that the range of performance was considerable. Five of the indicators analyzed had to be risk adjusted to account for variation in resident acuity among facilities. In 1997, Rantz and colleagues further described the process of verifying the accuracy of quality indicators derived from the MDS using four different methods: (1) structured participative observation, (2) a quality indicator observation scoring instrument, (3) independent observable indicators of quality instrument, and (4) survey citations. The research team was able to determine that quality indicators derived from MDS data did, in fact, differentiate nursing homes of better quality from those of poorer quality. Later work by Karon, Sainfort, and Zimmerman (1999) revealed that nursing home quality indicators are reasonably stable measures over short (3–6 months) periods of time.

The MDS and the Resident Assessment Instrument (RAI) continue to be examined for their usefulness in outcome measurement (Murphy, Morris, Fries, & Zimmerman, 1995–96; Fries et al., 1997; Mor et al., 1997; Phillips et al., 1997). The MDS and RAI constitute the foundation for monitoring the quality of nursing home care for case-mix reimbursement systems and for outcome-oriented long-term care research. Rantz and colleagues (1999) wrote that these assessment instruments improve care by identifying a resident's strengths and preferences as well as problems; they are used with an interdisciplinary approach; and they work best for clinical issues such as incontinence, impaired mobility, or skin breakdown. An AHCPR/AHRQ-sponsored study aimed at developing outcome measures in Massachusetts for the state's case-mix reimbursement system resulted in a set of resident outcome measures, including survival, functional status, continence status, pressure ulcers, and unplanned weight changes (Caro, 1995). In other research sponsored by the AHCPR/AHRQ, Spector and Fleishman (1998) reported that measures of functional disability play a key role in evaluating the outcomes of treatment.

Arling and colleagues (1997) conducted a project to develop a method for risk adjusting indicators of nursing home quality. Risk adjustment was implemented by stratifying residents into high-risk and low-risk groups and then calculating quality indicator rates within groups and drawing comparisons across facilities. Case-mix and other risk-adjustment methodologies are continually being evaluated in light of not only realistic measurement of outcomes but also new prospective-payment schemes. In the HCFA Multi-state Nursing Home Case Mix and Quality Demonstration Project, researchers analyzed data from four states and found significant differences in the quality of care even after risk had been taken into account.

In an article published in 1996, Lipowski and Bigelow explored data linkages for research on outcomes of long-term care by linking Medicaid claims with a sample of data gathered for nursing home quality-assurance and case-mix reimbursement. Resident records of the use of medical resources were combined with standardized assessments of health and functional status. The two data sources, one cross-sectional and the other longitudinal, complemented each other to provide a more complete description of not only health status but also use of resources.

One can examine quality indicators from three perspectives: (1) the resident versus facility level, (2) prevalence versus incidence of medical conditions, and (3) process versus outcome. At the resident level, quality indicators are defined simply as the presence or absence of a condition. Resident-level data can be aggregated across all residents in the facility to define facility-level indicators. At both resident and facility levels, a quality indicator that is defined as the presence or absence of a condition at a single point is referred to as a prevalence quality indicator, whereas a quality indicator that captures the development of the condition over time is called an incidence quality indicator. It should be noted that since comprehensive assessments are reviewed quarterly for each resident unless there is a significant change, prevalence may represent the prevalence of a condition over a three-month period.

Process quality indicators include those activities that occur between health professionals and residents (Hawes et al., 1997). Commonly, outcome quality indicators that are looked at as endpoints and outcome quality indicators refer to a change in current or future health status attributable to the care received. It is extremely important for researchers to revisit this outcome description in the long-term care setting, because it is more often relevant to consider the maintenance of health status as its own kind of outcome measure in nursing homes, where "recovery" is often not possible. Challenges include the need for continued work on risk adjustment as well as the determination of how to establish quality thresholds (Mukamel, 1997). For example, in comparing facilities, Zimmerman and colleagues (1995) suggested a threshold of performance equal to the 90th percentile of the state in which the facility exists.

A nursing home researcher should be familiar with generic outcome measures such as the SF36 Health Survey, the Quality of Well Being Scale, the Sickness Impact Profile, the Needingham Health Profile, and the Duke Health Profile. One of the most consistent findings in gerontological populations is the remarkable heterogeneity in functional status, emotional well-being, and health perceptions that is observed (McHorney, 1996).

Further work needs to be done on aggregating items in a set of quality indicators to form a meaningful composite score or index that can be used for comprehensive assessment of the quality of care in nursing homes (Heath, McCormack, Phair, & Ford, 1996a, 1996b). An important challenge raised by Hudson and Sexton (1996) is the difference in perceptions about priorities in nursing and health care. Hudson and Sexton collected their data in hospital medical-surgical units but raised an issue that should always be considered, particularly in a more consumer-driven system: to be sure that we understand what concerns and outcomes are most important to the patients and residents being served.

Rantz and colleagues (1999) have worked on a multidimensional theoretical model on nursing home quality integrating concepts such as the facility environment and philosophy, nursing and other staff, resident care, communication, and family involvement. Through the use of consumer focus groups, the model has been refined to reflect residents, families, staff, and community as central foci. In 2000, Rantz and colleagues began initial field testing of the Observable Indicators of Nursing Home Care Quality instrument.

Investigators in Oregon compared 38 assisted-living facilities ($n = 605$ residents) with 31 nursing homes ($n = 610$ residents) in terms of measures of residents' pain, psychological well-being, and activities of daily living. The researchers concluded that while residents in the assisted-living facilities were less disabled, the type of facility did not affect the resident outcomes over the year of study (Frytak, 2001). Landi and colleagues (2001) concluded that home care can prevent hospitalization, and a 1997 meta-analysis of 20 research studies by Hughes and colleagues revealed that home care can achieve cost savings in the care of the older population. However, the effectiveness of home care has still not been studied sufficiently.

In 2000, Dellefield conducted a review of the literature on the relationship between nurse staffing and nursing home quality. Higher total nursing staff levels are associated with functional improvement in residents, fewer medication errors, and fewer deficiencies. There is a positive correlation between higher staffing levels and not-for-profit status and a lower proportion of Medicaid residents. Anderson and McDaniel (1999) showed a positive correlation between RN participation in organizational decision making in nursing homes and improvement in resident outcomes. The use of Advanced Practice Registered Nurses in long-term care facilities improved outcomes in the areas of incontinence, pressure ulcers, and aggressive behaviors (Ryden et al., 2000). Staff stress in nursing homes is typically high owing to heavy workloads and caring for growing numbers of residents with dementia. A study of job strain in rural nursing homes by Morgan, Semchuk, Stewart, and D'Arcy (2002), showed that NAs had significantly more job demands than activity workers and were less likely than licensed nurses to perceive that they had enough time to do their work.

Grabowski (2001) looked at the effect of increasing Medicaid reimbursement on nursing home quality of care. Increased reimbursement improved care slightly. The quality measure used by Grabowski was the lower likelihood of a resident developing pressure ulcers. Despite progress in the long-term care health services research arena, the science is still young and incomplete and constitutes an important area for further development by researchers interested in long-term care.

MODEL PROGRAMS AND DEMONSTRATIONS

A major initiative to address the underutilization of nursing homes for both education and research was the five-year (1982–1987), $5 million Teaching Nursing Home Program funded by the Robert Wood Johnson Foundation. The purposes of the program were to improve the quality of clinical care in nursing homes, to create a conducive environment for formal graduate and undergraduate education as well as to promote the education of nursing home staff, and, finally, to encourage clinical research in long-term care settings previously underused as research environments. The teaching nursing home program, cosponsored by the American Academy of Nursing, established linkages between eleven schools of nursing and twelve nursing homes throughout the United States.

In 1997, Mezey, Mitty, and Vottrell published a follow-up study of the project to determine the enduring impact not only on the schools of nursing but also on nursing homes involved in the project. The deans and faculty of the eleven schools, faculty with joint appointments in both academic settings and collaborating nursing homes, and nursing home staff of the twelve nursing home facilities in the project were surveyed. The survey instrument addressed five areas: the durability of the affiliation between the schools and the nursing homes; the strengths and weaknesses of the teaching nursing home project; the most important educational outcomes as well as disappointments; factors in long-term viability of the model; and aspects of the project still in existence.

Mezey and colleagues found that the greatest impact of the teaching nursing home project on the quality of care in nursing homes resulted from the sharing of academic resources (i.e., the introduction of advanced practice nursing as well as faculty practice in general), consultation on the creation of special units, and an increase in clinical research. The teaching nursing home program had a role in the introduction of special care Alzheimer's units and the formation of ethics committees as well as in instituting and strengthening clinical policies, many of which remain in effect. Four clinical studies initiated during the teaching nursing home project were subsequently funded by the National Institute for Nursing Research. Interestingly, more respondents from schools of nursing than from nursing home staffs believed that the project led to lasting improvements in the quality of resident care.

Significant changes in clinical processes noted in the follow-up survey were decreased use of restraints and psychoactive medications, although it should be noted that these changes are also very likely related to the implementation of OBRA in the early 1990s. The outcomes of the teaching nursing home project included a reduction in the use of emergency rooms and re-hospitalization and an increase in behavior-management and incontinence programs (Mezey, Mitty, & Vottrell, 1997).

There were some innovative outcomes of the teaching nursing home project. A good example of innovation was the collaborative establishment of a long-term care institute by one nursing facility/school partnership that continues as an area resource to providers, regulators, consumers, and policy makers. A disappointment noted by nursing school and joint appointment respondents was the perceived resistance to changes in practice that seemed to be embedded in leadership issues. Relevant to the subject of research in nursing homes was the perception of communication problems between faculty and staff and the inability to engage and involve nursing home staff members in research. Specific concerns included resistance to changes in practice and the inability to sustain a commitment to innovation and research when there was a change in leadership. Chapter 5 details strategies for engaging staff members in research.

In 1994, despite a persistent dearth of literature that provided answers regarding quality improvement in nursing homes, nursing home providers in Wisconsin decided to put new ideas into action. An alliance of 11 nonprofit nursing homes initiated a quality improvement model known as Wellspring Innovative Solutions, Inc. The Wellspring model has six core elements: (1) an alliance of nursing home management committed to making quality of care a top priority; (2) shared services of a geriatric nurse practitioner (GNP) who provides leadership in the implementation of nationally recognized clinical practice models; (3) interdisciplinary care resource teams; (4) involvement of all departments within and across facilities in sharing best practices; (5) empowerment of all nursing home staff to make decisions affecting the quality of care and the work environment; and (6) continuous review of performance data throughout the Wellspring alliance. Key innovative components of the Wellspring model include the key role of the Advanced Practice Nurse, the GNP, and the attention to frontline staff. While preliminary analysis of the model is promising, and there is growing interest in replicating it, a more extensive evaluation is being conducted by the Institute for the Future of Aging Services at the American Association of Homes and Services for the Aging, with support from The Commonwealth Fund (Reinhard & Stone, 2001).

The Program for All-Inclusive Care of the Elderly (PACE) combines Medicare and Medicaid funding streams who are nursing home eligible, but whose care is a combination of home and adult day-care services. PACE had its origins in the San Francisco OnLok program in the early seventies. The philosophy is to maintain frail elders in their own communities as long as it is medically, socially, and economically feasible. The PACE model offers a range of integrated services delivered by an interdisciplinary team of providers (Eleazer & Fretwell, 1999; Boult & Pacala, 1999; Giacolone, 2001). The National PACE Association was formed in July, 1994, with quality assurance as its primary objective. Though client satisfaction in the PACE program is high, the number of enrollees remains small. A more recent approach is the Social Health Maintenance Organization, which involves an array of health and custodial services for Medicare beneficiaries who voluntarily enroll and pay a premium for services (Boult & Pacala, 1999; Giacalone, 2001).

SUMMARY

Nursing homes abound with opportunities for studying chronically ill older adults and for long-term health services research. Research in nursing homes, as with other segments of the health-care continuum, is increasingly focused on outcomes. The nursing home population is, by its very nature, high risk, and accurate risk-adjustment strategies continue to challenge nursing home researchers as well as financiers of nursing home care. In some ways, however, the nursing home industry is at an advantage, owing to a sophisticated national database that includes clinical data along with service delivery information.

Chapter 3

Ethical Issues
in Long-Term Care Research

Research ethics pose an impressive challenge for the long-term care researcher, as long-term care arenas are fraught with gray areas. For example, not only are nursing home residents generally frail, but also approximately 50 percent have some sort of dementia resulting in varying degrees of cognitive impairment. Hayley, Cassel, Snyder, and Rudberg (1996) described both ethical and legal issues prevalent in nursing homes owing to the complex physical and social conditions of residents and the myriad regulations in the industry. Frequently encountered issues include the implementation of advance directives, decision-making capacity and competence, and questions about the appropriateness of life-sustaining treatment, as well as risk management, the use of physical and chemical restraints, and the potential for abuse. The development of ethics committees and improved mechanisms for the protection of subjects participating in research are emerging trends. However, formal institutional review processes are often absent and other arrangements may be required (e.g., long-term care providers sign off on external institutional review board decision).

Through ethnographic analysis, Powers (2001) critically examined everyday ethical issues in nursing homes that are especially relevant owing to the high prevalence of dementia. She created a taxonomy of ethical issues, actually applicable to all long-term care settings, that included four domains: (a) learning the limits of intervention; (b) tempering the culture of surveillance and restraint; (c) preserving the integrity of the individual; and (d) defining community norms and values. The domains exist within the context of social values, individual values, and individual rights.

The preceding chapters addressed the relevance of research in long-term care and identified some interesting and timely research questions arising from the nursing home environment and, to a lesser extent, from assisted living and home care. However, the complexities of helping vulnerable subjects understand what it means to participate in a particular research study and protecting their rights to refuse or withdraw are enormous. Chapter 3 is intended to provide thought-provoking guidance for the protection of vulnerable research subjects. It entails a somewhat philosophical discussion along with some insights and practical guidelines.

FEDERALLY MANDATED RIGHTS FOR RECIPIENTS OF LONG-TERM CARE

The Omnibus Budget Reconciliation Act of 1987 included a Nursing Home Residents Bill of Rights, which formally and legally recognized residents' rights to:

- have free choice regarding treatment
- be free from restraints
- have privacy
- have confidentiality
- have their needs accommodated
- voice grievances
- participate in resident and family groups
- participate in other activities
- examine facility survey results
- refuse certain transfers within the facility
- have any other rights established by the U.S. Secretary of Health and Human Services.

The statements contained in this federally mandated bill of rights provide a backdrop not only for resident care but also for research endeavors in nursing homes. It is incumbent upon the nursing home researcher to uphold the bill of rights and to preserve residents' autonomy wherever possible in an environment in which many competing voices often attempt to speak on behalf of residents. In addition, the researcher must assure specific rights afforded to human subjects in the research process: informed consent without coercion, the ability to withdraw from participation in a research study without any negative ramifications, assurance of protection from harm and financial burden, and a guarantee to uphold dignity and privacy (Jaffe, 1999).

The Omnibus Budget Reconciliation Act of 1990 created a Home Care Clients Bill of Rights, which includes the following major provisions:

- The client must be informed of his/her rights, with the home health agency promoting and protecting them.
- Written notice of the bill of rights must be provided prior to initiating care.
- Agency compliance with the above must be documented in writing.
- The client, or the family or guardian in the case of a client whose decision making is impaired, can exercise the rights.
- The client has the right to have property treated with respect.
- The client has the right to express grievances regarding care, and the home care agency must investigate complaints made by the client, guardian, or family.
- The agency must provide information on advanced directives.
- The client has the right to confidentiality of clinical records, and the agency must advise the client of policies and procedures regarding the disclosure of records.
- The client has the right to be advised, prior to initiation of care, of expected payment by Medicare and other sources as well as the client's responsibility for payment.
- The client has the right to be informed of the toll-free home health care hotline in the state.

The principles contained in the home care bill of rights also provide a general backdrop for the ethical implementation of long-term care research in the home setting (Stackhouse, 1998). Fry and Duffy (2001) described the development and psychometric evaluation of the Ethical Issues Scale. Three components including end-of-life treatment issues, patient care issues, and human rights issues were demonstrated. In that same year, the American Nurses Association adopted a revised Code of Ethics for Nurses, including a mandate that the nurse promote, advocate for, and strive to protect the health, safety, and rights of the patient. Long-term care researchers would be well-served by adopting this mandate as a guiding principle.

Kapp (2000) raised the concern that research not conducted with federal dollars in nonacademic related long-term care settings may lack strong oversight from an Institutional Review Board (IRB) as mandated by the Office of Protection from Research Risks (OPRR) of the U.S. Department of Health and Human Services. He also raised the question of IRB accountability for the capacity assessment process that is addressed in succeeding sections of this chapter.

In 2002, the final medical information privacy rule of the 1996 Health Insurance Portability and Accountability Act (HIPAA) was published. HIPAA applies to health plans, health-care clearinghouses, and health-care providers transmitting health information in electronic form. HIPAA's definition of health care encompasses a broad array of care, services, or supplies related to health, including preventive, diagnostic, therapeutic, rehabilitative, maintenance, or palliative care and counseling. By definition, HIPAA affects the delivery of long-term care, including assisted living (Shelton, 2002). The final rule streamlined authorization requirements for research, permitting a single form to capture authorization to use protected health information as well as informed consent (Charters, 2003).

DECISION MAKING IN LONG-TERM CARE

McCullough and Wilson (1995, p. 10) addressed the general ethical and conceptual dimensions of long-term care decisions with the following thematic approach:

1. Decisions in long-term care are fuzzy and complex owing to the dynamics among the resident, staff, and family.
2. The process is not yet well understood, as principles of bioethics are borrowed from acute care.
3. Attempts to improve decision making in long-term care require challenging principles that dominate the bioethics literature.
4. Fresh approaches grounded in empirical studies and in the policy and historical contexts of long-term care are needed.

Long-term care decisions, couched in historically rooted institutional constraints, must reflect the appropriate limits on the exercise of professional power. In addition, rethinking basic concepts such as autonomy and independence, safety, and family roles and responsibilities is in order so that the orientation is toward a preventive ethics approach.

The vulnerability of subjects, in the context of who makes decisions regarding treatment, including experimental treatment, is a significant issue for the nursing home researcher. In defining vulnerable populations, one cannot make a case based on advancing age alone. However, increasing frailty and dependency, and often decreasing energy to make informed decisions, or decision-making capacity that is impaired by dementing illness, create the case for concern about vulnerability. Nursing home populations are, by and large, vulnerable. While value is placed on residents' rights to make choices, there is no gold standard for assessing decision-making capacity.

Some definitions are in order. *Incapacity* generally refers to a clinical determination of a person's inability to make an informed decision, whereas *incompetence* is a more formalized legal term for such an inability. In a clinical setting such as a nursing home, capacity and competence have autonomy as well as health-related "best interests, as their philosophical underpinnings." Decisional capacity is predicated on the possession of a set of personal values, the ability to communicate and understand information, and the capability of reasoning and deliberating about choices.

Principles and assumptions underlying the determination of decision-making capacity among older adults include: the constitutional right to make decisions regarding one's own life and well-being; the right to make decisions about health care treatment, including participation in clinical trials and other research initiatives; the right to be informed about health care options; and the right to set forth advance directives.

Mezey, Mitty, and Ramsey (1997) emphasized that decision-making capacity may not only fluctuate but also be unclear or, in some cases, completely and permanently impaired. The term "shades of incapacity" has been applied to these phenomena. Mezey and colleagues maintained that standardized mental status assessment tests may be insufficient to determine whether a person has the ability to make a specific health-care decision.

Smyer, Schaie, and Kapp (1996) explored the person-process-context dimensions of the ethics of decision making in later life. The person dimension involves the evaluation of capacity, whereas the process dimension entails ways of providing information. The context dimension involves engaging older adults, even when cognitive impairment is a factor. A later study by Kjervick, Weisensee, Anderson, and Carlson (1998) involved the development of instruments for measuring incapacity in the context of guardianship. A convenience sample of 206 subjects, including informal or family caregivers, health care professionals, and legal professionals, were asked to evaluate the content validity of 22 items related to determining incapacity. Of greatest importance were criteria related to the endangerment of self or others, and of least importance were criteria related to activity levels and social participation.

The work of Pruchno, Smyer, Rose, Hartman-Stein, and Henderson-Laribee (1995) suggested that the Mini Mental Status Examination, along with vignette-based measures for evaluation of decision making, could accurately determine the level of competency necessary to make treatment decisions in at least two-thirds of nursing home residents. Smith (1996) referred to the concept of negotiated consent, the elements of which are active participation by the patient and/or surrogate, at least a cursory knowledge of legal/ethical rights, and the opportunity for scrutiny and enforcement by a higher authority. Smith also identified the element of power in the deliberative process.

Another study in 1995 by Williams and Engle found that staff evaluation of competence correlated significantly with residents' scores ($n = 100$) on the Short Portable Mental Status Questionnaire. Staff members based their own assessments on orientation, alertness, and verbal function. Kapp (1994) recommended the development of institutional policies for assessing and documenting capacity.

Feinsod and Levenson (1998) proposed the following procedures for decision making, based on a framework of collaboration combined with the recognition of an individual's right to make and communicate his or her own decisions wherever possible:

1. Define the person's overall condition
2. Identify advance directive documents regarding personal wishes
3. Determine capacity and, if necessary, a substitute or proxy decision maker
4. Seek consultative support
5. Present options for consent

INFORMED CONSENT

There are four generally accepted elements of informed consent: informational elements including disclosure and comprehension, and consent elements involving competency and the ability to decide voluntarily. The actual process of obtaining informed consent involves three major components: (1) all relevant information must be conveyed; (2) the environment must be noncoercive; and (3) the patient or subject must be competent to make a decision on his or her own behalf.

The earliest use of a written consent form, as an application of informed consent, is thought to have occurred early in the 20th century. Truly informed consent, as the concept relates to research, involves communication about the proposed project: a project description, its purpose, the risks and benefits for the subject, the voluntary nature of participation and the freedom to withdraw, and alternative treatment options, if applicable (Cherniack, 2002).

A study published in 1996 by Barton, Mallik, Orr, and Janofsky determined the rate of incapacity to give informed consent for treatment among nursing home residents. Twenty of 44 newly admitted residents to a nursing home affiliated with a large teaching hospital were identified as incompetent to give informed consent based on the Hopkins Competency Assessment Test. Only 13 of the 20 were identified through staff observation as clinically incompetent. Barton and colleagues concluded that the prevalence of incapacity was high and that clinical screening failed to identify all of the incompetent residents. In the case of conflicting opinions regarding a resident's competence or in cases where competence is questionable, additional, more objective, testing is desirable and surrogate decision making may need to be explored. Weisenssee and Kjervik (2001) wrote that accurate assessment of cognitively impaired elders is a major policy challenge in an aging society.

Simmons and colleagues (1997) employed a screening rule based on four Minimum Data Set (MDS) indicators: cognitive patterns, communication/ hearing patterns, physical functioning and structural problems, and psychosocial well-being. Simmons and colleagues set out to determine the criteria for identifying residents who could accurately respond to yes/no questions about their care and thus participate in satisfaction surveys. Eighty-one percent of a sample of 83 nursing home residents was correctly classified using MDS indicators. The authors cautioned against ignoring individual differences even in the face of cognitive impairment. It is also useful to remember that competence is not unfluctuating in its properties; informed consent and the ability to participate in a study are somewhat related to the level of expectations.

SURROGATE DECISION MAKING

Surrogate consent comes into play when subjects lack the capacity to make an informed decision as to whether or not to participate in research investigations. Western society's dedication to autonomy has resulted in various laws and policies delineating the role of surrogate decision makers. Currently, two options exist for such decision making: the first allows a person, at a time when decision-making ability is still intact, a predetermined choice of another person who could make decisions, should it become necessary, through the execution of an advance directive; the second option addresses the assignment of an acceptable surrogate when there is no advance directive. In the absence of state surrogate legislation, this option involves the appointment of a guardian through the judicial system (Bosek, Savage, Shaw, & Renella, 2001). Unfortunately, less than 15 percent of the general population have written health care advance directives (Miller, Coleman, & Cugliari, 1997; Haynor, 1998).

Two key concepts underlie surrogate decision making: first, there needs to be a history between the surrogate and the person he or she represents; second, decisions should be based on knowledge of that person's needs, beliefs, and values. Therefore, surrogate or proxy decisions are to be based upon the incapacitated person's preferences and wishes, a principle often referred to as "substituted judgement." If preferences are unknown or unclear, the surrogate decision-maker must consider the other person's best interest (Bosek et al.). Typically, family members make the best choice for surrogates (Sprung & Eidelman, 1996).

Lynn (1992) wrote that all of us face the likelihood that at some point, usually in later life, we may be incapable of making informed decisions. Wicclair (1993) pointed out, however, that this situation is not unique to early or late life. Some people never acquire capacity, as is the case with developmentally disabled persons or when others lose capacity at various stages of life due to accident or illness. Health-related decisions, including choices regarding research participation, then must be made by proxy (with or without previous guidelines from the patient or resident), in advance by the patient, or through community and professional guidelines. Although the decision-making capacity necessary to appoint a health care proxy is less than the capacity needed to personally negotiate a living will or an informed consent, proxy decision-making is limited by the concern that proxies might act in self-interest or fail to mirror the patients' choice.

While surrogate decision makers are the best solution for making treatment decisions and for including persons lacking capacity in research, there are limitations to consider and respect:

• Difficulties separating the surrogate's needs from the patient's or subject's
• Complex and important decisions being made, often based on little specific guidance from the patient
• The surrogate being faced with decisions about treatment or research unavailable when the patient had decisional capacity
• Limited availability of the surrogate owing to distance or other commitments

• The surrogate's personal abilities and limitations and the willingness to assume responsibility. (Bosek et al.)

The following guidelines regarding surrogate consent, in the context of research, are adapted from Wicclair's work:

1. For research with therapeutic potential, surrogates may consent if, considering the nature of the proposed study and what is known about the subject, they can reasonably conclude that the person would have consented, or if they do not believe that the person would have refused to participate and participation is a sensible choice in terms of the subject's well-being.
2. For research without the potential of direct therapeutic benefit, surrogates may consent based on the nature of the proposed study and the conclusion that the person involved would have consented, or if they do not believe that the person would have refused to participate and the risks are minimal.
3. Whenever feasible, surrogate consent should be scrutinized by outside individuals (e.g., institutional review boards or ethics committees) who do not have a vested interest in recruiting subjects.
4. As the risks of participating in a study grow, the strength of the evidence supporting the conclusion that the subject would have consented must also increase.
5. Surrogate consent for research is acceptable only if the subject cooperates, signifying a form of assent.
6. All instructions given to surrogates and the criteria used in surrogate consent for a proposed study should be subject to review by an institutional review board.

In 1996, federal regulations governing research with human subjects were modified to allow for limited inclusion of unconscious patients in clinical trials of experimental drugs without the consent of patients or family, where relatives are unavailable. While this scenario applies primarily to patients with acute brain injury and thus would not be directly applicable in long-term care settings, the change in regulations has precedent-setting implications in terms of informed consent. The regulation addresses a situation in which the potential benefits of participating in a research protocol override consent requirements previously held sacrosanct.

Fost (1997) described the response of critics to the rule change. Critics argue that only a patient should decide whether or not to participate in an experiment, citing the first principle of the Nuremburg Code. The document drawn up by the Nuremburg Tribunal outlining principles by which to judge Nazi doctors' experimentation in concentration camps asserts that the voluntary consent of the human subject is absolutely essential. However, this principle has already been modified to encompass experimental treatment of children or incompetent adults. In such cases, health care experts, ethicists, and policy makers have broadly supported modified procedures allowing a relative to consent.

PROTECTION OF VULNERABLE SUBJECTS

Because advanced age is the primary risk factor for dementing illnesses such as Alzheimer's disease, there is an increasing likelihood of cognitive impairment as people grow older. Research into cognitive impairment and other common problems encountered in long-term care settings is a worthy endeavor, and nursing homes provide an accessible source of subjects. While a possible ethical rule, in the strictest sense, would be to allow no exceptions to personal consent, there are several limitations to such a rule. First, it denies the fact that at least some of the potential subjects who are cognitively impaired would choose to participate in research if they were capable of making an informed choice. Second, it limits access to possible benefits. Finally, even in the absence of immediate benefits to the subjects, it creates a barrier to evolving science (Wicclair, 1993).

According to Loue (2002), the National Institutes of Health acknowledge that cognitive impairment may render research subjects especially vulnerable, although U.S. regulations do not classify them as such. The NIH recommend the following considerations for conducting research with individuals who are cognitively impaired:

1. The consent process must clearly differentiate between accepted treatment and research.
2. The IRB should include at least one member who is independent of the proposed research project and has expertise in issues of decisional capacity.
3. Adequate assessment of participant capacity must be addressed in the research protocol.
4. There should be safeguards for additional protection of subjects as the severity of impairment increases.
5. Ongoing education should be conducted to enhance participant understanding.

6. Additional safeguards, such as the use of advanced directives for research, may be necessary when greater than minimal risk is involved. (National Institutes of Health, 1998)

The Alzheimer's Association has also recommended increased protection for subjects with diminished capacity, with the caveat that such subjects should not be prevented from participating in research. The association advocates that all individuals with Alzheimer's-related dementias be permitted to enroll in studies involving minimal risk, even if there is no direct benefit; that proxy consent be utilized in cases of greater than minimal risk but a reasonable potential of benefit; and that only those individuals still capable of giving informed consent or who have a previously executed advance directive for research be permitted to participate in studies involving greater than minimal risk and no direct benefit (Loue, 2002).

Certainly the whole issue of informed consent in vulnerable populations is a major challenge and may create a sticking point in the institutional review process. Obtaining informed consent in a nursing home can indeed be tricky and involves the cooperation of the administration, staff, and physicians or other health-care providers, as well as the residents and their families (Rapp, Topps-Uriri, & Beck, 1994; Sachs, Rhymes, & Cassel, 1993). It would be unfortunate to allow the challenges and difficulties of the consent process to stand in the way of much needed research.

THE POTENTIAL OF ADVANCE DIRECTIVES

One approach to the whole issue of informed consent is to address the matter formally through advance planning. Advance directives could address research participation specifically in a living will or through expressly empowering a proxy to make decisions about participation in research as part of health care decision making, as in a durable power of attorney for health care. The first condition avoids the necessity of evoking a standard of substituted judgment, and the second allows for choice regarding a trusted advocate.

The option of exercising advance directives was further legitimized by the federal Patient Self-Determination Act (PSDA) of 1991 (Teno et al., 1997a). The PSDA requires that all health care facilities receiving Medicare and Medicaid funding provide written information about advance directives. Advance directives include a living will or a patient's own declarations about wishes pertaining to decisions about health care with a focus on life-sustaining treatment. Advance directives also encompass health care powers of attorney, which are more flexible than living wills and more applicable to participation in research. Health care powers of attorney allow for choice in the selection of another individual or proxy to make a wide range of treatment decisions, not limited to life-sustaining treatments (American Association of Retired Persons, 1992). Actual legal forms and language vary from state to state, but the American Association of Retired Persons and the American Bar Association are good general resources regarding advance directives.

Teno and colleagues (1997b) evaluated the effect of advance directives on decision making as part of the Study to Understand Prognoses and Preferences for Outcomes and Risks of Treatments (SUPPORT). The investigators examined the content of the advance directive documents in the medical records of 569 subjects. Their findings revealed that advance directives did not guide decision making in the face of serious illness beyond naming a health care proxy (i.e., executing a durable power of attorney for health care or a health care power of attorney) or documenting only general preferences in a standard living will format. Even among the small number ($n = 36$) of subjects with specific advance instructions, actual care was often inconsistent with the directive.

Advance directives, particularly living wills, may not be comprehensive enough or may be written without adequate knowledge of the risks and benefits or potential lack of benefit of various treatment options. In a health care industry increasingly influenced by managed care concepts and cost constraints, aggressive treatment may be less and less likely to be covered financially. Furthermore, other barriers exist (e.g., communication, relocation) which interfere with any guarantee that an individual's wishes will be completely honored. Suri, Egleston, Brody, and Rudberg (1999) also found in a large-scale study ($n = 2,780$) that only a small minority of residents availed themselves of the opportunity to invoke care directives either before or after admission to a nursing home. The use of advance care directives was influenced by a number of demographic and functional characteristics. For example, older, Caucasian, long-staying residents were more likely to invoke advance directives. Residents with poor physical function were more likely to have self-generated care directives whereas those with impaired cognitive function were more apt to have only a physician-generated do-not-resuscitate order.

In the absence of an advance directive or appropriate proxy, community and professional guidelines become the last recourse. Such guidelines should reflect prevailing values and whatever information is discernible regarding personal preferences about a reasonable course of action in the face of uncertainty. Lynn (1992) proposed the following guidelines for authorizing or withholding treatment, guidelines that also have relevance for participation in research:

- formal and binding instruction directives for persons who have strong desires and want to settle matters in advance or who may have no logical proxy
- binding proxy directives, particularly when proxies are not the next of kin or otherwise obvious
- recognition of carefully considered oral directives
- a range of plans of care that are generally acceptable by community and professional standards
- the option for family and informal proxies to choose within the range with the oversight of collaborating health care professionals
- community responsibility for decision making for individuals with no proxies or specific advance directives through ethics committees, health care providers, or the legal system

The responsible and ethical conduct of well-designed research in long-term care settings is strongly supported by the American Medical Directors Association (AMDA), an organization of physicians serving long-term care facilities. However, a recent AMDA statement (2002) emphasizes that vulnerable subjects such as the residents of long-term care facilities, should be afforded full protection of both state and federal regulations concerning research in human subjects, regardless of the funding source and that, if anything, researchers need to exceed established standards. Key points of the statement included the following:

- Residents or their surrogates have the right to consent or refuse to consent to participation in research. Written informed consent must be obtained from subjects or their surrogates prior to participation in research projects.
- Consent to participate may be revoked by the subject or the surrogate at any time.
- Residents have the right to refuse to participate even when the surrogate has provided written consent.
- Research projects involving residents of long-term care facilities should be approved by both an external and internal institutional review process.

- The conduct of the research should be subject to continuous review.
- The risk of harm to participants should be low, and the potential benefits of the research should clearly outweigh the burden to participants.

Medical directors also asserted the right to approve a study before any subjects were enrolled, but that practice could be subject to debate in health services research and even clinical research involving nursing or social models. There are ethical dilemmas associated with "gatekeeping" practices when subjects, exercising their autonomy, desire to participate in research that has been through an institutional review process and does not affect medical treatment.

SUMMARY

Wicclair (1993) offered a comprehensive discussion regarding the application of research ethics to elderly recipients of long-term care. He wrote that even assent, or general agreement of a patient or resident to participate in a research study, is threatened by the influence of being in a dependent relationship and possibly by coercion and duress. In response to such potential threats, Wicclair initially suggested two options: to avoid conducting research without therapeutic potential, and to avoid conducting research in agencies that have a history of regulatory noncompliance or questionable care practices. Wicclair's own analysis of the first option challenges it by asserting that exploratory and descriptive long-term care research provides important scientific knowledge to a variety of disciplines and often ultimately promises at least indirect benefit. Participation in any sort of research methodology can also provide an enjoyable diversion for individuals who serve as subjects.

As in all matters of ethics, the application of research ethics in a long-term care environment is laced with gray areas. For example, research ethics in nursing homes will always remain embedded in personal values, concern for residents' dignity, and concern for the protection of a population that is, for the most part, dependent and vulnerable. Researchers will encounter legal and regulatory issues, end-of-life issues, limited resources, and the challenge of involving staff members who are largely paraprofessionals (Kane, 1995a). Best practices are not always clear because, while the literature is replete with information about the ethics of long-term care, there is a paucity of information specifically applicable to research. However, at the very least, the savvy researcher will tailor consent information to the needs of the chronically ill, allow additional time for review, incorporate multiple assessments of competence, and involve the family in the research process.

Chapter 4

Issues of Research Design in Long-Term Care

Particularly in light of the changing demographics of society, both nationally and globally, perhaps no health-related issue is capturing more attention than long-term care. Perhaps no other health issue is as important or as complex. Researchers seeking to establish the best methodologies for addressing the complexities of long-term care may wish to heed the words of Edwin Land, "Don't undertake a project unless it is manifestly important and nearly impossible."

Despite the good news about general improvements in health status in the elderly, a growing prevalence of chronic illness is anticipated, with a concomitant increase in the need for long-term care and assistance with basic self care and activities of daily living, instrumental activities of daily living, and even the maintenance of social interaction. These anticipated trends will require data-driven clinical innovations and education, increased funding, and creative public and private programs (Anderson, 2002). We will be challenged to orient federal programs toward community-based long-term care and monitor the quality of such care. These changes will require enhancing support to family and other informal caregivers. Continuous improvement in the quality of institutional care is needed. All of the challenges will require new ways of thinking about increasing the supply of highly skilled long-term care workers (Rantz, Marek, & Zwygart-Stauffacher, 2000; Cubanski & Kline, 2002).

Research in long-term care is needed to guide public policy, owing to the following issues and problems:

- The long-term care system is fragmented.
- Consumers are often subjected to multiple assessments in the determination of the appropriate level of care.

- The availability of long-term care services varies widely.
- There is an evolving long-term care workforce crisis.
- There is still a lack of consensus in how to measure long-term care quality.
- Efforts to ensure long-term care quality have been largely punitive.
- Problems persist with funding and reimbursement for long-term care services. Despite Medicaid waivers for community-based long-term care, an "institutional bias" persists.
- Development in community infrastructures to support a long-term care continuum is needed.
- A comprehensive long-term care database at the state and national levels needs further development for long-term care policy analysis. (Silberman et al., 2002)

Long-term care research, then, should encompass several domains: clinical research that seeks to improve the treatment of individuals with chronic health problems; the testing of models for enhancing quality of life, satisfaction for patients, family, and staff, and other psycho-social-spiritual aspects of long-term care; consumer participation in establishing preferences and involvement in care management, and continued study of quality long-term care regarding organizational and financing arrangements, including the interface of external assessments such through regulatory surveys and accreditation processes.

DESIGN AND METHODOLOGY

Research in long-term care generally fits within the realm of applied research, i.e., research for the purpose of seeking new knowledge to drive long-term care solutions as opposed to basic research that seeks knowledge for the sake of knowledge. Clinical trials are designed to improve the treatment of chronic health problems and improve overall health status through examination of the effects of clinical interventions. Clinical trials typically involve a descriptive-correlational or experimental design, with research in long-term care settings being no exception. Descriptive correlational methods seek to determine relationships between variables, without manipulating variables as part of the investigation. An experimental design, on the other hand, entails manipulation of one or more variables. The effects of the manipulation of the experimental (independent variable) on the outcome (dependent variables) are measured in experimental research.

This kind of research, especially in environments such as long-term care settings, is often actually quasi-experimental. In other words, it is impossible to assure a controlled environment, in terms of extraneous variables and it is difficult to meet other rigors of a true experimental design, e.g. random selection and assignment of subjects. Unfortunately, many clinical trials in long-term care are conducted with small samples, or never replicated. To be relevant, clinical research dissemination and application in the form of practice guidelines are necessary. More studies on improving care for people with chronic conditions with existing treatments as well as comparative studies examining the effects of new treatments and technologies need to be supported (Eastman, 2002).

Research regarding the psychosocial aspects of long-term care, quality of life issues, and satisfaction with care often is conducted using a descriptive or exploratory approach. Investigators seek to gain useful information to inform directions in long-term care, without examining specific relationships or treatment effects. Kane (2001) wrote that long-term care, especially in nursing homes, is often balanced toward technical quality, but not quality of life. Research in quality-of-life domains—security, comfort, meaningful activity, relationships, individuality, autonomy, dignity, privacy, functional competence, and spiritual well-being—is sparse and confusing. While the limited research on consumer preferences in long-term care reveal a widespread aversion to nursing homes among community-dwelling elders, nursing home residents typically demonstrate a relatively high level of satisfaction. In 2001, Kane and Kane attempted to piece together roughly 20 years of sporadic research, using interviews, questionnaires, and focus groups as data collection techniques. Aspects of care that have been shown to be important to nursing home residents include kindness, caring, compatibility, and responsiveness. Residents value control, choice in their daily lives, and privacy, along with competent care. Elders receiving long-term care at home also value competence as well as compatibility with their care providers, reliability, respect for their preferences, and adequacy in the amount of help received. In a larger sense, they look for physical, social, and psychological outcomes and quality processes, as well as reliability, honest, and integrity.

In June of 2000, the Board of Directors of the Association of Health Services Research, now the Academy for Health Services Research and Health Policy adopted a new definition of the field of health services research, reflecting its growing sophistication and continuing evolution: "Health services research is the multidisciplinary field of scientific investigation that values how social factors, financing systems, organizational structures and processes, health technologies, and personal behaviors affect access to health care, the quality and cost of health care, and ultimately our health and well-being. Its research domains are individuals, families, organizations, institutions, communities, and populations" (Lohr & Steinwachs, 2002, p. 8).

Health services research actually encompasses a range of basic to applied research. A variety of methods are employed in the health services research arena, including descriptive designs, e.g., retrospective review of medical records and secondary analysis of existing databases. While experimental designs in clinical research measure the effects of patient interventions, these methods are also applied in health services research to measure outcomes associated with changes in health-care delivery. Findings can then be used to formulate data-driven health policy. A health services approach is used to evaluate quality of long-term care programs. According to a 2001 report by the Institute of Medicine, defining or evaluating quality of long-term care is an impressive challenge. While we have national databases of systematic information about nursing homes, for most other settings, systematic data is nonexistent or very limited and lacking in uniformity. There is little agreement about what constitutes quality as much of the available information is open to interpretation and conclusions are not based on empirical evidence. Three specific features of long-term care are relevant for assessing quality: first, long-term care is both a health program and a social program; second, the potential and actual role of consumers is an essential element of long-term care; and third, the physical environment in residential care facilities and nursing homes plays a role in quality as it contributes to privacy, physical safety, mobility, and, in a larger sense, to quality of life.

Community-based long-term care research methodologies are affected by the fact that patients in the community tend to be less homogeneous than in residential settings. However, frailty results in a certain degree of commonality among patients such that research may produce less than dramatic results in terms of measurable improvements in health status. On the other hand, more promising results may be obtained through efforts to maximize quality of life and avoid declining life satisfaction (Weissert & Hedrick, 1999). Nursing home research offers more homogeneous populations to study, but there is an even greater conundrum about the appropriateness of various interventions in terms of cost/benefit ratios and a general lack of consensus regarding the desired outcomes of intervention. There is concern about not only the further development of practice guidelines, but also about the stability of the long-term care workforce to assure implementation (Schnelle & Reuben, 1999).

SAMPLING

Sample selection in clinical long-term care research involves some prediction of which subjects stand to benefit from enhanced or altered clinical treatment. However, on the basis of demographics alone, it is important to enroll more long-term care subjects in clinical trials (Eastman, 2002). Sampling strategies used in other health care settings also apply in long-term care, and involve projecting the desired sample size and determining how the sample will be drawn. The long-term care researcher must choose from various sampling strategies such as convenience sampling, cluster sampling, random sampling, and stratified sampling techniques. The process may involve sampling medical records as opposed to human subjects.

Enrolling subjects and maintaining a sample in long-term care settings are challenging at the very least. There are several strategies for enrolling potential subjects. Key informants in the nursing home, including administrators, directors of nursing, charge nurses, and social workers, initially can help to identify potential subjects. To be most efficient, the informants must have a clear understanding of the inclusion and exclusion criteria for the study so that they don't identify unsuitable residents. In addition, a thorough chart review is useful, although the records may vary, making it difficult to obtain consistency. For example, if inclusion criteria for a study include "cognitive impairment," the medical record may not provide sufficient information to establish the existence and nature of the impairment. There may be several different ways that any sort of criteria are characterized in the records. For example, cognitive impairment may be indicated by dementia, confusion, chronic brain syndrome, or organic brain syndrome.

The next step after identifying potential subjects through informants or record review is to develop efficient, nonintrusive screening procedures. Initial screening may be done before obtaining informed consent to conserve time and resources. In some cases, this can be as simple as the ability to state one's name, address, telephone number, and/or age and birth date. Potential subjects may also be asked to repeat the purpose of the study and what will happen to them during the course of the study. For a more comprehensive evaluation to determine ability to give informed consent, the Blessed Dementia Scale (BDS) may be used to determine degree of cognitive impairment. The BDS is a 17-item screening instrument that is a holistic, objective measure which is completed by caregivers rather than the subject. It contains items that measure everyday activities, and has been found to be sensitive and specific as a screening test for dementia as well as for activities of daily living and transitional health status (Blessed, Tomlinson, & Roth, 1968; Mohs, 1987; McDougall, 1990).

In the screening process, it is important to attempt to determine whether a resident is able to adhere to a research protocol. However, screening measures do not always accurately portray a subject's ability to comply. To overcome this limitation, the "run-in strategy" has been used for some nursing home research studies. The run-in strategy gives potential subjects practice in all or part of the study before randomization. Subjects are eliminated from the study if they demonstrate poor adherence during the run-in (Lang, 1990). For example, a run-in strategy was employed by Ouslander and Schnelle (1993) to determine whether nursing home residents were able to participate in an incontinence protocol. Potential subjects were placed on a toileting program for a one-day run-in period, and data were collected relevant to their ability to answer prompts about wetness and dryness and their ability to toilet. The data accurately predicted residents' ability to be responsive to a toileting program over longer time periods, although this technique involves some risk of selection bias.

Another challenge in nursing home research is obtaining a large enough sample for the generalizability of the findings. Some constraints for obtaining an adequate sample are difficulties in obtaining informed consent, failure of residents to meet study eligibility criteria, and attrition. In an NIH-funded Harvard Teaching Nursing Home project, 53–82 percent of 700 potential subjects were excluded from various studies, and only 14–81 percent of those eligible consented to participate (Lipsitz, Pluchino, & Wright, 1987). In many cases, several nursing homes must be used either to attain an adequate sample size or to prevent contamination between treatment and control groups within a site. A problem with using multiple sites is the issue of variability among nursing homes. One way to address this issue is to assess the nursing home environments with the Multiphasic Environmental Assessment Procedure (MEAP) to ensure that they are as homogeneous as possible. The MEAP contains five scales, which measure physical and architectural features, policies and programs, resident and staff characteristics, social environment as perceived by residents, and observer-noted environmental quality. The MEAP has been administered in over 200 nursing homes, and normative data, reliability and validity are established for each scale (Moos & Lemke, 1984; Lemke & Moos, 1987).

Once the subjects have been enrolled, the next challenge is maintaining the sample. Some reasons for subject attrition are clearly beyond the investigator's control, such as change in physical or cognitive status, illness, hospitalization, transfer to another facility, and death. Attrition rates can range from 15 percent to 20 percent or more during a six- to twelve-month time period (Gloth & Burton, 1990; Langer, Drinka, & Voeks, 1991; Kunin, Douthitt, Dancing, Anderson, & Moeschlberger, 1992; Rapp, Topps-Uriri, & Beck, 1994; Matteson, Linton, Cleary, Barnes, & Lichtenstein, 1997). Oversampling based on previous studies with similar populations, pilot studies, or descriptive statistics from the previous year in the nursing home or homes in which the study will take place is the most efficient way to deal with these types of attrition.

In other cases, attrition can be associated with factors that are generally within the investigator's control, such as nursing home staff attitudes or a change in the attitude of the subject or family. Because of their close proximity, staff members can strongly influence subjects' and family members' participation in research projects. Staff members must believe that the research is important and that the research is not detrimental to the residents. The staff members must be thoroughly educated about the research protocol before and during the study. In addition, it is helpful for the investigator and/or research associate to be in frequent contact with the staff members to exchange feedback and to provide positive reinforcement. Meetings with staff can be on an individual basis or in a group setting.

DATA COLLECTION

A long-term care researcher may want to avail himself or herself of information contained in three major national data systems, including:

1. The On-line Survey Certification and Reporting (OSCAR) System is a computerized database of survey and certification information for Medicare and Medicaid-certified long-term care facilities. It provides information on regulatory performance, resident characteristics and conditions, facility characteristics, staffing, and complaints.
2. Currently, data from the Resident Assessment Instrument (RAI) are being electronically entered into a national database.
3. The Outcome and Assessment Information Set (OASIS) is a group of data elements representing core items of a comprehensive assessment of adult home care patients. It is one key focus of Medicare's partnership with the home care industry to foster and monitor improved home health outcomes.

Anderson, Madigan, and Helms (2001) referred to the federally mandated OASIS as an information revolution in home health care. The authors cited the potential for meaningful, scholarly inquiry to be enhanced by the standardization and electronic transmission of patient information. They challenged researchers to:

• Test the reliability and validity of OASIS items
• Explore the dynamics of information sharing in home care
• Investigate how information systems can be used by staff to prioritize and deliver patient care

Data collected directly from recipients of long-term care or from staff providing care requires careful planning and selection of data collection techniques and instrumentation. A number of instruments have been referenced elsewhere in this book, but oftentimes the administration of instruments has to be adapted for long-term care populations. New instruments may need to be developed, a process that itself involves data collection. For example, Sorlie, Sexton, Busund, and Sorlie (2001) used self-ratings of patients and ratings of clinicians in developing a global measure of physical functioning, then went on to test the psychometric properties of the instrument. A compilation of issues and instruments regarding satisfaction of both consumers of long-term care and long-term care staff was developed by Cohen-Mansfield, Ejaz, and Werner in 2000.

New research questions may benefit from initial exploratory work, using a qualitative approach. Unstructured interviews and focus groups are useful techniques in trying to understand phenomena that have not been studied. Qualitative data, in turn, may be incorporated into instrument development. Triangulation, or the use of multiple methods of data collection, often produces the richest results.

FUTURE ISSUES IN LONG-TERM CARE RESEARCH

Schnelle and Reuben (1999) suggested three emerging forces in nursing homes that will require further study: (1) the effects of regulatory efforts on organizational change; (2) appropriate use of clinical practice guidelines; and (3) the impact of changing financing structures, such as managed care, on the ability to improve outcomes while controlling coats. The Wellspring Model (Reinhard & Stone, 2001) adds further detail to a future research agenda for nursing homes, recommending further work in:

• Developing and implementing model systems of practice
• Establishing internal quality assurance systems

- Strengthening nursing home staff
- Improving the regulatory process
- Modifying Medicare and Medicaid reimbursement

Walshe (2001) asserted that for a variety of reasons, nursing home regulation isn't working very well. However, as a necessary step in improvement, research is needed to better understand the reasons for its failings.

The formulation of good science in long-term care will require cross-disciplinary thinking and studies of individuals in an organizational context as well as how the organization tends to the needs of individuals. Jared Diamond (1999) began his popular work on the history of different cultures' material success, with a question raised by Yali, a young man from New Guinea, "Why is it that you have so much cargo, when we have so little cargo?" (p. 14). In 2002, Phillips adapted Yali's question to query, "Why are some nursing homes better than others?" Phillips goes on to validate that accumulating the knowledge necessary to answer Yali's question will require continuing quantitative work regarding models and variables, complemented by qualitative investigations. Qualitative approaches should focus on developing a better understanding of the interaction between organizational cultures, structures, and processes, and the long-term care products and outcomes.

In 2002 Joanne Handy, President and CEO of the Visiting Nurse Association of Boston and Chair of the Board of the American Society of Aging, Joan Quinn, Senior Vice President of Blue Cross and Blue Shield of Connecticut, Mary Alice Ryan, Chair of the Board of the American Association of Homes and Services for the Aging, and Josh Wiener, Principal Research Associate at The Urban Institute, shared their predictions for long-term care for 2010. They each highlighted the evolving trend of providing long-term care in the least restrictive environment. These experts predicted further expansion of home and community-based services, driven by demographic changes, consumer demand, technological advances, and efforts to achieve greater economic effectiveness. Russo (2002) underscored the 21st century role of technology in process management, clinical interfaces, interactive and remote monitoring, and data collection and analysis in home care. Benjamin (2001) posed issues for further exploration in long-term care services delivered at home, querying how consumer-directed services at home can be flexible, responsive, and cost effective, while meeting the standards of accountability for publicly-funded services. Watt (2001) also challenged that the sheer numbers and longevity of noninstitutionalized elders invites a potential health delivery crisis. She suggested an interdisciplinary program such as a community-based case as a model for outcome-based research. In 2000, the editors of the journal *Home Care Provider* provided long-range expectations of industry experts, which also addressed the role of technology as well as changing reimbursement schemes, greater accountability, and preventive services such as nutrition interventions in the elderly.

Additional research is needed in transitional care environments that bridge acute and long-term care. We need to identify patients who would benefit most from these kinds of services, to determine the nature and intensity of services needed to achieve the most desirable outcomes, and the type and level of providers needed to deliver the care. Also cost and access components need further study, comparing and contrasting existing and emerging models of transitional care (Naylor & Prior, 1999).

Other research questions actually arise out of the research process itself in long-term care settings. For example, issues surrounding the informed consent process beg questions such as "are elders less informed, or are there widespread alterations in judgment in the population receiving long-term care, that threaten the integrity of the process?" (Cherniack, 2002). Actions that facilitate the skills of surrogate decision-makers need to be tested and outcomes and issues associated with reliance on surrogates need to be examined (Bosek et al., 2001).

SUMMARY

This chapter has actually set the stage for conducting long-term care research, starting with some background issues for consideration, and continuing with making decisions about design and methods, which of course is driven by the nature of the research question and existing knowledge of the topic. Sampling and data collection issues are discussed. Finally, a conceptual discussion of future issues affecting long-care is included to provided a contextual framework for research in long-term care.

Chapter 5

Gaining Access for Research

This chapter focuses on the many challenges to gaining access to long-term care settings, particularly nursing homes, for the purposes of conducting research. The first and major challenge is dealing with the mistrust, skepticism, and threat that the nursing home administration, staff, residents, and families frequently feel about research. The same kind of skepticism and feelings of vulnerability exist in other long-term care settings; however, the complexity of these issues is probably greatest in nursing homes.

Nursing home administrators are concerned about the perceived value of the research, the welfare of the residents, and the potential costs of the research to the nursing home resulting from requirements for supplies and space, disruption of the care routine, and other increased demands on staff time. Concerns may relate to other factors such as the added responsibilities involved in preparing and transporting residents to research activities, identifying surrogates and witnessing informed consent, providing information on behavioral and functional status, answering questions from residents and families, and assisting with the administration of treatment protocols and the assessment of outcomes. There is also typically concern about the issue of research protocols conflicting with regulatory requirements, and even fear of possible litigation as nursing homes are frequently targets of lawsuits by family members.

There is often tension between researchers, who are typically academicians and perceived as working in "ivory towers" as opposed to the real world of the nursing home. The nursing home staff may be threatened by outsiders who are observing their care routines, as well as by the possibility that the research may lead to more work. Because nursing home residents are a vulnerable population, nursing home staff and residents' families may feel a need to protect the residents from experimentation or possible exploitation. The staff may be skeptical about the ability of research to improve the care of very old, frail, and severely impaired residents. The risk-benefit ratio for the residents and their families, as well as the nursing home administration and staff, is a real concern. If the study seems to have no immediate benefits for the residents or the institution, and benefits only the researcher and/or society in general, the usefulness and feasibility of the research may be questioned.

The specific types of challenges faced by investigators depend on the research questions and methodology. The majority of published long-term care studies are descriptive rather than experimental. As discussed in Chapter 4, descriptive studies are primarily related to health-care services research, and the methodology involves gathering data through medical records review, observations, interviews, or questionnaires. These studies generally are carried out to evaluate the quality of care; staff retention and resource issues; administration, efficiency, costs, and outcomes of care; resident characteristics, morbidity and mortality; family caregiver issues; and legal issues. Access to records and subjects, as well as the use of supplies and space, are the major challenges in gaining access for descriptive studies.

Experimental studies involve clinical trials or interventions for residents, families, or staff members. In addition to many of the challenges encountered when gaining access to conduct descriptive studies, experimental studies present even more formidable challenges, which may account for their scarcity in the literature. Clinical trials or intervention studies generally involve some type of program evaluation in which either the staff members are taught to carry out various interventions (Schnelle, McNees, Crooks, & Ouslander, 1995; Beck et al., 1997) or trained interdisciplinary teams implement the interventions (Kartes, 1996; Przybylski et al., 1996; Ray et al., 1997; Slaets, Kauffman, Duivenvoorden, Pelemans, & Schudel, 1997) or, in some cases, trained research assistants carry out the research protocol (Koroknay, Werner, Cohen-Mansfield, & Braun, 1995; Steffen & Mollinger, 1995; MacRae et al,, 1996). Some studies involve a combination of these practices (Evans et al., 1997; Matteson, Linton, Cleary, Barnes, & Lichtenstein, 1997). Case managers actually delivered the intervention in a home care study by Landi and colleagues in 2001. In addition to access to records and subjects, a fundamental challenge in experimental studies is gaining the cooperation and approval of the administration, staff, and subjects to carry out the intervention. Investigators must convince the institution that disruption of the care routine, and the number of tasks involving preparing and transporting residents to research activities, identifying surrogates and witnessing informed consent, providing information on behavioral and functional status, answering questions from residents and families, using supplies and space, assisting with the administration of treatment protocols, and assisting with the assessment of outcomes will be minimal for the employees.

Generally, whether the studies are descriptive or experimental, the more time, work, and cost of the study that the investigators take upon themselves, and the fewer additional demands on the staff and administrators, the more likely the acceptance into a nursing home.

STRATEGIES FOR GAINING ACCESS

The first step in gaining access to nursing homes for research purposes is to educate nursing home administrators, staff, and residents' families regarding the significance of the study and the benefits of the research to the institution and residents. The study should be scientifically sound and clinically relevant, and should include safeguards for the safety and confidentiality of subjects, having undergone review by the appropriate Institutional Review Board. Administrators and staff members are more receptive to research if the study addresses ongoing clinical problems and if the interventions are feasible in typical nursing home settings. If the protocol has the potential to benefit the individual residents who participate (rather than nursing home residents in the future), residents, families, and staff members will be more receptive than if the benefit is not immediately tangible (Ouslander & Schnelle, 1993; Ryden et al., 2002).

Nursing home administrators, staff, and residents' families also must be assured that the risks of participating in the study are minimal. In general, the risks should be no greater than those the nursing home resident might incur in everyday life, including invasive and noninvasive procedures such as physical assessment, mental status testing, functional assessment, medications, and urinary catheterization.

It is useful to conduct a pilot study before carrying out a major research project in a nursing home. A pilot study provides information about the feasibility of gaining access to the subjects' medical records, collecting data, implementing treatment, involving staff members in the protocol, and evaluating outcomes. Preliminary data also help identify potential dropout rates and justify sample sizes, allowing for the appropriate rates of attrition.

The following sections are organized as step-by-step, "how to" guides:

Meeting With System Representatives and Administrators

First, meet with the nursing home administrators, including the executive officer of the particular nursing home conglomerate, and the individual nursing home administrators, nursing and medical directors, and charge nurses. When everyone is involved during the early stages of the development of the protocol, many misunderstandings can be avoided and cooperation is more likely. Researchers must first develop a good relationship or rapport with the administrative staff. The administrators are the gatekeepers of the institution, and their cooperation is essential for a successful study.

Establish a cooperative rather than adversarial relationship. Reducing the threat to the institution and its stakeholders is essential. They must be assured of the study's purpose and that the study will be a cooperative venture among the facility, the staff, the residents, their families, and the researcher. It helps to acknowledge the value and worth of the facility, its employees, and its residents.

It is helpful to seek administrators' input into the study protocol as it is being developed. They have a "real world" view of the possibilities for research and can point out barriers to carrying out the protocol and suggest ways to increase the feasibility of implementation. Because researchers have a reputation for having an "ivory tower" view of nursing home care and practice, spoken of previously, this is an opportunity for researchers with clinical expertise to demonstrate their real world knowledge or for researchers who have been away from the field for awhile to gain this type of knowledge. A dialogue with the administrators can strengthen the study protocol.

Inviting administrators at all levels to be "research associates" on the project encourages "buy-in" and ownership of the study. One study included all of the key administrators as either research associates or consultants on the grant proposal. Depending on their contributions, they were included in paper presentations and given credit for being a part of the study. This strategy ensured full cooperation of the institution.

Clearly delineate the roles, responsibilities, time commitments, and resources of everyone involved in the study from the beginning. Administrators must know exactly who will be responsible for specific tasks as well as the time involved in carrying them out, and should give their explicit approval and support.

Demonstrating the benefits of a study may pose different challenges for researchers who are conducting descriptive research and those who are carrying out experimental intervention studies. Investigators who are obtaining data from medical records for epidemiological studies regarding such items as demographics, costs, record keeping, and adherence to regulations may have a difficult time convincing nursing home administrators that there would be any benefit to their allowing access to records. In addition, descriptive studies involving staff, residents, or family members, such as observing staff-resident interactions or asking staff, residents, or family members to fill out questionnaires or participate in interviews, may seem time consuming and of no benefit to the participants, as opposed to intervention studies.

There are several ways to demonstrate the benefits of a study. The first is to verify that the information gained from the study may lead to further studies that will directly benefit the administration and staff. For example, if a researcher discovers that the record-keeping methods are excessively time consuming for the facility, a follow-up study may test methods that may be more efficient. The researchers also may inform the administrators that the information gained may lead to cost-cutting measures, lower staff turnover, and higher quality of care, especially if several nursing homes are involved in the study and unique or creative ideas are found in the other nursing homes that could be adapted for use in the particular facility. Finally, the fact that a research project is being conducted in a nursing home may be a source of pride to administrators at both the local and the system levels. Some chains of nursing homes as well as individually operated facilities advertise that they are part of ongoing research to benefit the operations of the system and the institution. A researcher may point out to administrators that other nursing homes find this to be a benefit rather than a disadvantage.

Owing to the fact that negative press and public perception are relatively common phenomena, nursing home administrators have many fears about their facilities being exposed as they often are in the media, as places where the cost is high, care is poor, and residents are abused. When researchers enter a nursing home and examine the operations of the facility "under a microscope," administrators may feel threatened, both from an institutional and personal perspective. Egos become involved, as well as other issues such as power, control, and intimidation (researchers with advanced degrees can be quite intimidating). One researcher who was conducting a descriptive study of residents with dementia was barred from looking at the residents' records by a person who was in charge of the area Medicaid office. Although the nursing home was under the oversight of the Medicaid office, the official was not involved in the everyday administration of the nursing home. The official's reason for banning access to the records was to protect the residents' privacy, even though permission had been given through approval by an Institutional Review Board and the administration of the nursing home. This situation appeared to be a power issue, but the Medicaid official allowed the study to proceed after the researcher changed an innocuous sentence in the consent form to the official's liking. The researcher had to make the extra effort to have the changes in the consent form approved by the human subjects committee, and the delays brought about by this incident held up the study significantly.

The researcher must convince administrators that all information obtained will be completely confidential, both within and outside the facility. The concept of confidentiality is well known to researchers who are obtaining approval for the study through granting institutions; however, long-term care administrators may not be comfortable with assurances of confidentiality. Administrators must be certain that they or their agency will not be exposed in any negative way.

Good communication skills and humility on the researcher's part are the keys to allaying administrators' fears and securing successful entry into the system. Remember that the researcher is a guest in the nursing facility and should treat everyone in the facility with courtesy and kindness—just as a guest would treat hosts in their home. Mutual respect is a key ingredient for success; arrogance and pomposity have no place in this situation or environment.

While many of the same principles for gaining access for research apply to the home care setting, the Association for Home Care Web site contains a feature very useful to researchers—an agency locator with contact information. Many state level home-care associations offer the services and advice of a research committee and a history of receptivity to research. Hospital-based agencies may fall under the umbrella of the hospital's institutional review committee and/or ethics committee. Having a professional advisory board is a condition of Medicare certification. It is incumbent on the researcher or research team to educate those individuals in the administrative structure and the home-care staff as well as patients and families regarding the benefits of the study and the protections for patients (Sherry Thomas, personal communication, February 4, 2003).

Working With the Staff

It is essential for the researcher to meet with all of the staff members who will be involved in the research protocol. The supervisor of the unit involved in the study can act as a liaison between the staff and the administration, and should be included in both administrative and staff meetings. (Clinical studies should include the director of nursing and the medical director.) Many researchers have had the experience of having the full cooperation of the administration, and then, when the study begins, meet with resistance from the staff members who were not included in the early planning.

The type and degree of staff involvement depend on the methodology of the study. For descriptive studies, it may mean helping gain access to information in the subjects' medical records, nurses' staffing reports, or accounting reports from the business office. It could also mean participating in interviews, answering questionnaires, or being observed during care. For experimental studies, staff members may be taught to carry out the protocol, or may work with the research assistants who are carrying out the protocol, or both.

In this heavily regulated industry, the staff may fear close scrutiny in relation to record keeping, caregiving, and communicating with one another, residents, and families. The care that nursing personnel provide is labor intensive, and the problems of inadequate training, understaffing, low pay, and staff turnover contribute to stress, shortcuts, and short tempers. In addition, the nursing assistants who provide most of the hands-on care may feel that their observations and suggestions for care are not valued. A researcher must do everything possible to allay their fears about strangers invading their territory and assure them that the information gained will be strictly confidential and will not jeopardize their jobs.

Staff members may be concerned about the additional work involved, particularly in intervention studies. One way to address this is to tell them that there may be additional work now, but knowledge gained from the study may lead to less work later on. Another is to tell them that learning to carry out the proposed clinical protocols may actually decrease work immediately, because the protocols may produce more efficient ways of providing care. In addition, some clinical trials investigating new medications and treatments may reduce the incidence of symptoms of disease or promote healing more quickly, resulting in the rewards of seeing residents' health status improve and ultimately less work for care providers.

When explaining the purposes and methods of the proposed study to the staff, it is useful to be simple and concrete. The nonprofessional staff members may be intelligent, but not highly educated, especially with regard to the research process. Rather than lecturing to them, involve them in discussions of their observations and the problems they have encountered to gain their interest and ownership of the research project. Treat them with the same respect with which the administrators are treated, and acknowledge their value as care providers.

When staff members themselves are the subjects in a study, they must be assured that all the information they give will be anonymous or confidential.

Interviews or questionnaires that they fill out may contain sensitive information regarding their feelings about the institution, administration, other staff members, residents, or family members. Staff members tend to be suspicious about answering questionnaires. In one study, the questionnaires were placed in large, brown envelopes that were coded so that the information was anonymous, with no means of determining who the respondents were. One respondent wrote on the questionnaire, "You say this is anonymous, but I know you know who I am, and I won't answer the questions. I know what I say will get back to my supervisor." An investigator must develop alliances with members of the staff and act as an advocate rather than as an adversary.

Meeting With Residents and Family Members

Nursing home residents and their family members are involved as subjects and/or informants and are crucial to a clinical research study. Subjects may worry about what will be done to them and whether their dignity or privacy will be violated. They may fail to see the benefit of participating in a research project, refusing to be "guinea pigs." Conversely, many residents welcome the attention and the opportunity to contribute to science and possible improvements in nursing home care.

Gaining residents' consent to participate in research studies has been discussed in earlier chapters, but the process can be problematic when subjects have difficulty with vision and/or hearing, so their understanding of the nature and implications of the study may be limited. The situation is further exacerbated for residents with various levels of dementia. Residents should be assessed for mental status so that a determination of competency can be made. When they are not competent to give informed consent, consent must be gained from a family member or guardian. In any case, researchers should always attempt to obtain either oral or written "assent" to participate from the residents in order to have the fullest possible cooperation.

Family members may be asked to give permission for the residents to participate in the study. They may be very skeptical about the research process, and need to be apprised of the balance of risks and benefits of the study, particularly for frail nursing home residents who are at the end of life. Comfort issues are uppermost in their minds, and they appropriately want to protect their aging family members from any undue distress. Sometimes they may agree to participate for altruistic reasons (i.e., it may not benefit my parent or spouse, but the lessons learned may benefit others).

Family members themselves can be the subjects of study, through answering questionnaires or participating in interviews, observation, or possibly some type of intervention. Having to place an aging relative in a nursing home can be stressful and may lead to feelings of guilt, anger, grief, relief, or myriad other feelings. For these reasons, family members may refuse to participate in a study or, conversely, may welcome the opportunity to express their feelings to an objective listener or observer. They may even consider this an opportunity to share with others the knowledge they have gained from the experience.

COMMITMENT TO SHARE RESULTS OF THE STUDY

Most nursing home administrators, staff, residents, and family members are more willing to consent to participate in a study if they are assured that the results of the study will be shared with them, regardless of the outcomes. A formal presentation may be made to the nursing home employees as well as resident subjects and/or family members. An oral report is preferred over a written report so that there is the opportunity to discuss the findings and to assess the impact that the study had on the subjects and nursing home employees. Negative results may be presented in a positive manner by pointing out the benefits of gaining such knowledge, and sensitive results can be judiciously shared with nursing home administrators, who may want to decide how they are presented to the employees, subjects, and/or family members. All participants also must be assured that any presentations or publications of the results will not reveal the identity of the institution or its constituents.

SUMMARY

Chapter 5 has detailed a pragmatic, step-by-step approach to gaining access to nursing homes for the purpose of conducting research. Like many other types of health-care agencies, the nursing home system is often an organization with complex structural dynamics. There are formal (administration) and informal (staff) power structures that must be acknowledged when the study is being developed and when cooperation is sought at all levels. The nursing home researcher must engage administrators, staff, residents, and families in the research process by minimizing threats, creating buy-in to the project, and building excitement about the journey toward the development of useful new knowledge. The following approaches are useful in promoting communication and gaining the cooperation of administration and staff:

- Gain support from formal power structures during the development of the study
- Gain support from informal power structures to maintain their support and commitment throughout the study
- Conduct meetings and actively negotiate with administration and staff members to keep them informed and involved in the study throughout the process
- Establish ground rules and clearly delineated roles for the research protocol

Researchers must be cognizant of the major issues involved in the early stages of a research project, including understanding the nursing home system and its sociopolitical structure, and communicating with administration, staff, residents, and family members. The discussion of gaining access for research has focused on nursing homes as the most complex and highly regulated of long-term care settings. However, the principles and "how to" guidelines presented here are generally applicable to other residential long-term care settings, as well as home health care.

Chapter 6

Implementing Long-Term Care Research

The implementation of a research study can be a lesson in problem solving and troubleshooting. To preserve the integrity of the study, it is helpful to anticipate problems and attempt to prevent them from occurring. When problems do occur, it is helpful to have strategies formulated for solving them beforehand to prevent a precipitous deterioration of the protocol.

Implementing a research project in a nursing home requires some special considerations. Phillips and Van Ort (1995) discussed the influence of selected factors on research in long-term care and how such factors may threaten internal validity, and suggested some ways of minimizing such threats. One of the sociopolitical factors they identified was that, over time, the nursing home staff developed images and myths about residents that defined the residents and how much could be expected of them. Images are positive in that they help to individualize care; however, images can be a barrier when researchers set out to implement interventions that require a new behavior for a resident, or that otherwise violate the staff's images or basic assumptions. The resulting staff reaction (protectiveness) may interfere with the progress of the study.

The power dynamics in long-term care are often complex. Formal power rests with professionals who may spend little time with residents or other staff members, but who shape the behavior of the nonprofessional staff. The informal power structure among the nonprofessional staff rests to a great degree on their personal characteristics and the longevity of a few individual staff members. The influence of informal power is strong and not always congruent with the goals of the formal power structure. In addition, one must overlay the influences of individual family members and residents. Most nonprofessional staff members in long-term settings are not well educated and have a limited number of care-management strategies within their knowledge base. There may be issues resulting from low socioeconomic and occupational status, including health problems, lack of transportation, family problems, and a perceived lack of dignity or internal rewards on the job (Phillips & Van Ort, 1995). To engage the staff's interest in research and their commitment to a successful research project, the researcher must understand and appreciate these issues.

Phillips and Van Ort also suggested the following strategies for minimizing threats to a study's internal validity and for ensuring the overall success of a nursing home based research project: gaining support from formal power structures early in the study period; conducting meetings with all relevant staff members to reach consensus on the ground rules of the research protocol; keeping the staff informed and involved with the project; working with informal power brokers to maintain their support and commitment; and actively negotiating with the staff, as necessary, throughout the process.

Whoever is charged with the direct conduct of a study must develop a close working relationship with the administration, staff, residents, and families. It can be bothersome to nursing home employees to have an extra person on the unit who is collecting data from medical or nursing records or disrupting the regular care routine by collecting data from residents. For example, a data collector may have all the charts out in the nurses station—taking up room, using charts that staff members may need, or simply being a nuisance. A place for the data collector to work and store files should be prearranged to avoid conflict.

One strategy that has been successfully used by a research associate to promote cooperation was to provide occasional snacks for coffee breaks for the staff as a means to thank them for their participation and to meet with them in an informal setting. A research associate who is on site frequently can develop an excellent working relationship with the staff, and they can become loyal supporters of the study. Residents and family members who have a positive relationship with the research associate are more likely to cooperate as well. They all need to feel that a researcher in any capacity is an advocate rather than an adversary.

Both formative and summative evaluations are important as the study is being conducted. Periodic meetings with the staff, administration and family members are useful for ongoing progress reports and exchange of information. When the study is completed, it is extremely important to report the findings to all participants, including administrators, staff members, subjects, and/or family members. In addition, when appropriate, the names of the "research associates" in the nursing home should be included in paper presentations or publications. If a clinical intervention was tested and successful, the staff members are more likely continue to carry out the protocol after the study is completed. They are generally proud to have assisted in the development of a model of research-based care.

CLEARLY DELINEATED ROLES

When a researcher enters the long-term care setting, either to conduct a descriptive or an experimental study, his or her role must be clearly defined. This is especially true for researchers with clinical backgrounds. Staff members frequently consider a person who is in the research role to be in a position to render direct care or to provide consultation. This can be frustrating for staff members, patients or residents, and families when needs arise and the researcher cannot respond to these needs. According to Patterson (1994), several strategies can facilitate the process of establishing and maintaining the role of researcher in a nursing home:

- *Define the researcher role.* Clearly defining what constitutes the role of the researcher for that particular study before entering the setting helps to avoid potential difficulties in later maintaining this role.
- *Establish clear boundaries.* Depending on how the researcher role is defined, the degree of involvement with the staff members and residents may vary. Some studies may involve implementing direct care as an essential aspect of the methodology, whereas others may involve participant observation. In the latter situation, achieving a balance between the role of participant and the role of observer is critical.
- *Allow adequate time for entry.* Allotting sufficient time to become familiar with the setting promotes the establishment of relationships essential to setting the tone for the study.
- *Consult with others.* Maintaining open communication with administration and staff members provides feedback regarding the impact of the researcher's presence on the staff members and may help to prevent potential difficulties.

IDENTIFYING AND ADDRESSING CHALLENGES

The most frequent challenges encountered in long-term care research are enrolling subjects and maintaining a sample; obtaining accurate information from medical records; and carrying out various tests or interventions with requirements for specialized equipment, space, or staff cooperation. Many factors are out of the control of the researcher, but they must be addressed to successfully complete a study. The challenges of enrolling subjects and maintaining a sample are described in Chapter 4. Using medical records in long-term care settings can also be a challenge as they may be lacking in information necessary for collecting research data. Medical evaluations and diagnoses can be scanty, abbreviated, and incomplete, and the reliability and validity of nursing information have not been well established. The most valid and reliable information is related to administration of medications because of strict requirements for documentation. Researchers generally use the records for screening purposes only, and then perform their own data collection specific to their needs.

The formatting and content of records can vary considerably from one agency to another, making it difficult to obtain data that have adequate reliability for comparisons. The Minimum Data Set (MDS), a federally mandated assessment instrument, helps to provide consistency in reporting various aspects of the health and well-being of residents. The MDS helps to ensure standardized, accurate information and provide a clear definition of content areas that are being rated.

Data collection procedures can become quite cumbersome in long-term care environments. Researchers are generally left to their own devices when specialized tests are involved, and they usually must either import equipment or transport subjects to another location. In many cases, research protocols must be modified because the testing is too expensive or impractical.

Administration of questionnaires, physical and functional assessments, and other types of assessments may require a specified space or quiet area for testing. In many residential facilities especially, space is scarce, and securing an appropriate environment may be difficult. Older people should be tested in an environment that promotes their comfort and ability to communicate easily. As was illustrated in Chapter 1, residents in a nursing home population generally have at least one chronic illness and are usually functionally and/or frequently cognitively impaired. Variability in the day-to-day functional abilities can cause variability in assessment results. In addition, sensory deficits and cognitive impairments can lead to environmental distractions that can contaminate test results. Every attempt should be made to ensure an appropriate setting for assessment and testing. The researcher may have to end a testing session and return several times to ensure valid data collection.

To better understand methodological challenges associated with intervention research in nursing homes, Hershey, Collins, Gershon, and Owen (1996) reviewed two studies aimed at reducing back injuries among nursing home staff and two studies aimed at preventing occupational transmission of blood-borne pathogens. Based on their review, Hersey and colleagues emphasized that research projects are strengthened by adapting rigorous designs to the real-world setting of the nursing home, by employing multiple measures to detect effects, and by communicating findings to policy makers.

In a clinical trial, the interventions are carried out by either the researcher or research assistant, or by the nursing home staff. If the researcher is performing the intervention, it is helpful to determine the feasibility of carrying out the intervention and the extent to which staff assistance is available. For example, an inexperienced researcher conducted a study to determine whether group reminiscing would decrease levels of depression. The researcher found a quiet room in which the group could meet, scheduled weekly sessions at 10 A.M., but assumed that the staff would assist by making sure the subjects were ready and helping transport them to the session. The morning of the first session, most of the subjects were still in bed and hadn't gotten dressed, and it soon became apparent that they could not be gotten up in time for the session. When it appeared that this would be an ongoing phenomenon, the sessions were rescheduled for immediately after lunch when the residents were already up and in the dining room; the group leader transported them to the room where the intervention was to take place. Although the procedure was extremely time consuming, it was the best way to ensure attendance at the reminiscing sessions. In addition, the "quiet" room had an intercom system, and periodic announcements distracted the group participants. One of the participants who was hearing impaired thought that an announcement was a page for him, and he stood up and started to leave the session. The group leader spent a great deal of time trying to persuade him to stay until the session ended. Many of these problems can be forestalled if a researcher anticipates them by developing a relationship with the staff, and by becoming familiar with the routine, the structure, and the everyday functioning of the nursing home.

When staff members are charged with carrying out a clinical trial, the researcher must take special care to ensure that the protocol is followed. Education of staff members, careful oversight of the interventions, and particular attention to documentation are crucial to the success of the study. Either the researcher or research assistant must be on site to oversee the details, troubleshoot and problem solve. The researcher needs to maintain excellent communication skills and interpersonal relationships, be creative and flexible, have good problem-solving skills, and be well acquainted with the long-term care environment, as described in Chapter 1. In the design and implementation of a restorative model for home care, the researchers and professional staff collaborated with home health aides to identify and pilot test solutions (Baker, Gottschalk, Eng, & Tinetti, 2001).

It may happen that at least one member of the administration or staff is uncooperative with the investigation or the researchers. Sometimes promises of support are made when the project is being developed and there is lack of follow through after the study begins. For example, in one study, the goal was to withdraw subjects from their psychotropic medications while a behavioral intervention was implemented to decrease problematic behavioral symptoms of dementia. When the study protocol was being developed, the medical director of the nursing home had agreed to be a research associate in charge of the drug withdrawal protocol in consultation with a geriatrician who was a co-researcher. However, when it came time for the medication withdrawal, the medical director resisted, expressing concern for the residents and staff if agitated behaviors increased. After many reassurances that the subjects would immediately be put back on medications if behaviors became unmanageable and in consultation with the co-researcher, he finally agreed to the drug withdrawal protocol. (Incidentally, the behavioral symptoms decreased.) In the same study, a staff nurse refused to implement the protocol claiming it was "ridiculous," and with all of her experience, she knew best how to care for dementia patients. When the researcher determined that nothing would change her mind, she was simply omitted from the project. However, as the study proceeded, the researcher asked for her input and provided positive reinforcement for her skills as a nurse. Toward the end of the project, she finally was convinced that the methods of the study had some merit and she became fully cooperative, even claiming ownership of the research project.

EDUCATING STAFF MEMBERS

Investigators can employ several strategies to ensure that everyone receives the education necessary for implementing the study. It is generally useful to have informal group sessions that allow for give and take between the leader and the participants. An exchange of ideas is important to determine the needs of the staff members and their level of understanding. It is very difficult to gather staff members together, so several sessions are necessary. One of the best times to gather the participants is at the change of shift. Staff members can come early or stay late before or after their shift when they are free of their caregiving activities. Teaching videotapes can be made for the staff to view. The researcher or research associate can keep attendance, answer questions and determine whether the staff has gained the knowledge that they need through return demonstrations. Paper-and-pencil tests also can be given. Staff members can be asked to view all of the tapes before participating in the implementation of the study. Any new staff members also must be educated about the study and the protocol. Showing the videotapes is a useful way to ensure that as each new staff person is employed and participates in the protocol, the education is completed.

According to Lekan-Rutledge (2000), difficulties in implementation of research protocols occur most often when the following barriers exist:

• Inadequate numbers of staff
• Inadequate staff communication and support
• Inadequate initial education of all involved staff
• Lack of ongoing education and reinforcement
• Insufficient monitoring of implementation
• Failure to select appropriate subjects
• Failure to evaluate progress

Incentives and rewards for cooperation and participation in a research study are necessary for satisfactory staff involvement. Individual verbal feedback and praise are essential. Other rewards such as awarding pins and certificates, commending employees to their supervisors, and giving public credit for participation within the framework of presentations and publications of the research create a feeling of pride in the research and related accomplishments. For example, pins may be awarded that say "Research Unit" to each staff member upon completion of the educational component of the project. Sometimes they may be awarded individually and other times they may be presented in a special ceremony for a small group of people. The pins denote caregivers as special, marking them as integral participants in the project and promoting a feeling of ownership in the research study.

Again, many of the same principles for implementation of a research study apply to the home care setting. HIPAA standards also provide privacy protections for information gathered using the OASIS assessment instrument. Perhaps the most unique difference to which the researcher needs to be sensitive lies in the fact that in this kind of care delivery, care occurs strictly on the patient's turf. There also tend to be more extraneous variables to consider in this very uncontrolled setting (Sherry Thomas, personal communication, February 4, 2003).

AFTER COMPLETION OF THE STUDY

As noted in Chapter 5, investigators have an obligation to follow up with all of the research participants after the study is completed. Presentation of the findings, public acknowledgment, kudos and thank you's, and feedback and evaluation should be shared with everyone involved in the study. These opportunities promote partnerships with nursing homes for future collaboration, and in the case of successful clinical trials, may inspire the ongoing and continued use of the protocol for improved care of the nursing home residents.

It is useful to award certificates to every person who participated, including administration, staff, residents, and family members. A reception may be held during which participants can be honored and thanked. The participants can derive great satisfaction from knowing that their important contributions have been acknowledged, opening the door for further research in the nursing home. Following an investigation regarding management of dementia, the involved nursing homes continued to provide care using the research protocol, citing it as a model of care for residents with dementia.

SUMMARY

Successful implementation of a research project in a long-term care setting involves clearly delineating the roles of the researchers and staff, strategies for screening and enrolling subjects and preventing attrition, access to medical records, and ongoing staff education. Recognition of anyone involved in carrying out a research study to completion is a critical part of the process.

It is possible to change clinical practice in the setting where the study is conducted as well as in other long-term care settings. The best way to change behaviors is to convince long-term care personnel that the clinical intervention has been successful and has resulted in beneficial outcomes for the individuals for whom they provide care. The intervention must have a "real life" application and must make sense to the staff for them to believe in it and adopt it as practice. In addition, the staff members need to have ownership in the study and to be rewarded for their contributions.

Chapter 7

Dissemination of Findings

New knowledge gained through long-term care research can help to address the many challenges of chronic care. However, nothing useful is achieved unless research findings see the light of day, i.e., are published or otherwise put into the hands of those who can effect positive changes in the delivery of long-term care. The intended audience includes policy makers and administrators, staff, and even residents and their families.

Mueller and Cam (2002) cited several barriers to adoption of research-based protocols in long-term care, including staffing shortages, inconsistent patient assignments, lack of knowledge and lack of enthusiasm regarding protocols, difficulty changing routines, and complex organizational cultures, particularly in nursing homes. Nursing homes that are early adopters of innovations tend to be larger facilities with chain membership and a higher saturation of private pay residents (Castle, 2001).

Dissemination begins by sharing the results of the study with the participants, students, and colleagues at a national and/or international level. It involves giving credit to appropriate people in both presentations and publications. This is not only an ethical issue, but also ensures that the nursing home and others will be more open to research at their facility in the future. When appropriate, research associates at the facility should be named as co-presenters for the study.

In the long-term care arena, it is critical that research findings be disseminated to policy makers, with a special emphasis on health services research findings. In 2001, Feldman, Nadash, and Gursen posed the following questions:

- What types of research do policy makers draw on for strategic policy development?
- What are the critical gaps in knowledge from the perspective of long-term care researchers versus policy makers?

95

- What makes an effective information broker?
- What actions can be taken to better address the dissemination of long-term care research and the effective translation of findings for policy makers?

From the perspective of policy makers, the source of information matters and the substance matters. In addition, the translation, the format, and the timeliness matter.

How do long-term care researchers assure that research findings reach the audiences who can change the practice of long-term care? The findings from clinical studies in particular need to be put in the hands of clinicians to empower them to engage in research-based practice. State and national association meetings (e.g., the American Health Care Association, the Association of Homes and Services for the Aging, the National Association for Home Care, and the Assisted Living Association), and newsletters are excellent avenues for the dissemination of findings. There are a number of journals that publish long-term care research, including highly referred geriatric research journals, such as the *Journal of the American Geriatric Society*, *The Gerontologist*, and the *Journal of Gerontology*. There are also journals specific to the long-term care industry such as *Annals of Long Term Care and Nursing Homes* for nursing home audiences, and in the home care arena, *Home Health Care Management and Practice*, *Home Health Services Quarterly*, *Home Care Provider*, *Hospice Journal*, and *Home Health Nurse*.

Manuscripts submitted for publication need to be written clearly and according to the guidelines and style requirements of the target publication. However, in addition to poor writing quality, manuscripts are rejected for many other reasons according to Sullivan (2002):

- There is not a good fit between the manuscript and the journal.
- The manuscript content does not provide new information.
- The information is out of date.
- The topic is too narrow or appeals to a narrow audience.
- Out of date references are used or other important contributions to the topic are missing.
- The author has relied too heavily on related literature.
- Too little information about the methodology is given, or the methodology contains serious flaws.
- The manuscript does not make a clear point.

Additionally, scientists need to be able to describe their work and must be skilled in explaining it to clinicians who have not had extensive research training and to the public. Chappell and Hartz (1998) recommended presenting or writing about a scientific discovery as a detective story for lay audiences. Communicating research in this way also means paying attention to a factor known as the Fog Index, or diminuation of clarity, which is determined by analyzing words and sentence length, and roughly estimates the amount of formal schooling required for understanding written work. Writing for the general media, another important avenue for disseminating research findings, especially to the public, necessitates such considerations. The general rule of thumb is to target individuals with an eighth-grade education.

It has been said that if research has not been disseminated and published, it hasn't been conducted. The results of a study need to be disseminated widely, not only to other researchers and to clinicians, but also to consumers and policy makers. Long-term care policy is a huge issue, both at state and federal levels. Long-term care settings provide a rich environment for research because subjects are long-staying in a self-contained, circumscribed, potentially controllable environment. Consequently, there is the opportunity to investigate many problems amenable to intervention, particularly over time. However, the conduct of long-term care research presents many challenges. Researchers must be cognizant of the major issues involved, including understanding long-term care systems,especially the nursing home system and its sociopolitical structure; communicating with administration, staff, patients, and family members; and using strategies for carrying out research protocols successfully.

References

Aaronson, W. E., Zinn, J. S., & Rosko, M. D. (1994). Do for-profit and not-for-profit nursing homes behave differently? *Gerontologist, 34,* 775–786.

Agency for Health Care Policy and Research. (1997). *AHCPR research on long-term care.* Silver Spring, MD: Author.

Ahronheim, J. C., Mulvihill, M., Sieger, C., Park, P., & Fries, B. E. (2001). State practice variations in the use of tube feeding for nursing home residents with severe cognitive impairment. *Journal of the American Geriatrics Society, 49,* 148–152.

Allen, J. E. (1999). *Assisted living administration: The knowledge base.* New York: Springer Publishing.

American Association of Retired Persons (1992). *A matter of choice: Planning ahead for health care decisions.* Washington, DC: Author.

American Health Care Association (1999). *Facts and trends: The nursing facility sourcebook.* Washington, DC: Author.

American Health Care Association (2001). *Staffing of nursing services in long term care: Present issues and prospects for the future.* Washington, DC: Author.

American Medical Directors Association (2002). Protecting clinical trial participants in nursing facilities. *Caring for the Aged, 3*(4), 1, 22.

Anderson, G. F. (2002). Nurses prepare for the growing numbers of persons with chronic conditions. *Nursing and Health Policy Review, 1*(1), 51–61.

Anderson, M. A., Madigan, E. A., & Helms, L. B. (2001). Nursing research in home health care: Endangered species? *Home Care Provider,* December, 200–204.

Anderson, M. A., Wendler, M. C., & Congdon, J. C. (1998). Entering the world of dementia: CAN interventions for nursing home residents. *Journal of Gerontological Nursing, 24*(11), 31–37.

Anderson, R. A., Hsieh, P. C., & Su, H. F. (1998). Resource allocation and resident outcomes in nursing homes: Comparisons between the best and the worst. *Research in Nursing and Health, 21,* 297–313.

Anderson, R. A., & McDaniel, R. R. Jr. (1998). Intensity of registered nurse participation in nursing home decision making. *Gerontologist, 38,* 90–100.

Anderson, R. A., & McDaniel, R. R. Jr. (1999). RN participation in organizational decision-making and improvements in resident outcomes. *Health Care Management Review, 24*(1), 7–16.

Arling, G., Karon, S. L., Sainfort, F., Zimmerman, D. R., & Ross, R. R. (1997). Risk adjustment of nursing home indicators. *Gerontologist, 37,* 757–766.

Baker, J. J. (2000). *Prospective payment for long-term care 2000–2001.* Gaithersburg, MD: Aspen Publishers, Inc.

Baker, D. I., Gottschalk, M., Eng, C., & Tinetti, M. E. (2001). The design and implementation of a restorative model for home care. *The Gerontologist, 41,* 257–263.

Banaszak-Holl, J., & Hines, M. A. (1996). Factors associated with nursing home staff turnover. *Gerontologist, 36,* 512–517.

Barton, C. D. Jr., Mallik, H. S., Orr, W. B., & Janofsky, J. S. (1996). Clinicians' judgment of capacity of nursing home patients to give informed consent. *Psychiatric Services, 47,* 956–960.

Beck, C., & Chumbler, N. (1997). Planning for the future of long-term care: Consumers, providers, and purchasers. *Journal of Gerontological Nursing, August,* 6–21.

Beck, C., Heacock, P., Mercer, S. O., Walls, R. C., Rapp, C. G., & Vogelpohl, T. S. (1997). Improving dressing behavior in cognitively impaired nursing home residents. *Nursing Research, 46,* 126–132.

Benjamin, A. E. (2001). Consumer-directed services at home: A new model for persons with disabilities. *Health Affairs, 20*(6), 80–95.

Berglund, B., & Nordstrom, G. (1995). The use of the Modified Norton Scale in nursing-home patients. *Scandinavian Journal of Caring Sciences, 9,* 165–169.

Bergstom, N., & Braden, B. (2002). Predictive validity of the Braden Scale among black and White subjects. *Nursing Research, 51,* 398–403.

Bergstom, N., Braden, B., Laguzza, A., & Holman, V. (1987). The Braden Scale for predicting pressure sore risk. *Nursing Research, 36,* 205–210.

Billipp, S. H. (2001). The psychosocial impact of interactive computer use within a vulnerable elderly population: A randomized prospective trial in a home health care setting. *Public Health Nursing, 18,* 138–145.

Binstock, R. H., & Spector, W. D. (1997). Five priority areas for research on long-term care. *Health Services Research, 32,* 715–730.

Blaum, C. S., Fries, B. E., & Fiatarone, M. A. (1995). Factors associated with low body mass index and weight loss in nursing home residents. *Journal of Gerontology, 50A,* M162–68.

Blessed, G., Tomlinson, B. E., & Roth, M. (1968). The association between quantitative measures of dementia and of senile change in the grey matter of elderly subjects. *British Journal of Psychiatry, 114,* 797.

Bliesmer, M. M., Smayling, M., Kane, R. L., & Shannon, I. (1998). The relationship between nursing staffing levels and nursing home outcomes. *Journal on Aging and Health, 10,* 351–371.

Bond, G. E., & Fiedler, F. E. (1998). The visibility of organizational culture in a long-term care facility. *Journal of Nursing Administration, 28*(4), 7–9.

Bosek, M. D., Savage, T. A., Shaw, L. A., & Renella, C. (2001). When surrogate decision making is not straightforward: Guidelines for nurse administrators. *Journal of Nursing Administration's Healthcare Law, Ethics, and Regulation, 3*(2), 47–57.

Boult, C., & Pacala, J. T. (1999). Integrating care. In E. Calkins, C. Boult, E. H. Wagner, & J. T. Pacala (Eds.), *New ways to care for older people: Building systems based on evidence.* New York: Springer Publishing.

Bowers, G. (2000). The future of home care. *Home Care Provider, February,* 18–24.

Branch, L. G. (2001). Community long-term care services: What works and what doesn't? *The Gerontologist, 41,* 305–306.

Brooks, S. (1996). What's wrong with the MDS? *Contemporary Long Term Care,* November, 41–47.

Bruck, L. (1997). Welcome to Eden. *Nursing Homes,* January, 29–33.

Caro, F. G. (1995). Health outcome measurement in nursing homes. *AHCPR Research Activities, 204,* 19.

Castle, N. G., & Banaszak-Holl, J. (1997). Top management team characteristics and innovation in nursing homes. *Gerontologist, 37,* 572–580.

Castle, N. G., & Fogel, B. (1998). Characteristics of nursing homes that are restraint free. *Gerontologist, 38,* 181–188.

Castle, N. G., Fogel, B., & Mor, V. (1997). Risk factors for physical restraint use in nursing homes: Pre- and post-implementation of the Nursing Home Reform Act. *Gerontologist, 37,* 737–747.

Castle, N. G., Mor, V., & Banaszak-Holl, J. (1997). Special care hospice units in nursing homes. *Hospice Journal, 12*(3), 59–69.

Castle, N. G., Zinn, J. S., Brannon, D., & Mor, V. (1997). Quality improvement in nursing homes. *Health Care Management: State of the Art Reviews,* June, 39–54.

Castle, N. G. (2001). Innovation in nursing homes: Which facilities are the early adopters? *The Gerontologist, 41,* 161–172.

Centers for Medicare and Medicaid Services (2001). *Appropriateness of Minimum Staffing Ratios in Nursing Homes.* Report to Congress prepared by Abt Associates, Inc., Cambridge, MA.

Chappell, C. R., & Hartz, J. (1998). The challenge of communicating science to the public. *The Chronicle of Higher Education,* March, 87.

Charter, K. G. (2003). HIPAA's latest privacy rule. *Privacy, Politics, and Nursing Practice, 4,* 75–78.

Chattopadhyay, S., & Ray, S. C. (1996). Technical, scale, and size efficiency in nursing home care: A nonparametric analysis of Connecticut homes. *Health Economics, 5,* 363–373.

Chen, C. C., & Cohen, S. S. (2002). Rooms without rules. *Policy, Politics, & Nursing Practice, 3,* 88–97.

Chenier, M. C. (1997). Review and analysis of caregiver burden and nursing home placement. *Geriatric Nursing, 18,* 121–126.

Cherniack, E. P. (2002). Informed consent for medical research by the elderly. *Experimental Aging Research, 28,* 183–198.

Chiu, L., Shyu, W. C., & Liu, Y. H. (2001). Comparisons of the cost-effectiveness among hospital chronic care, nursing home placement, home nursing care, and family care for severe stroke patients. *Journal of Advanced Nursing, 33,* 380–386.

Cleary, B. L. (1992). Life in a nursing home. *Abstract in Proceedings of International Council on Women's Health Issues,* Copenhagen, Denmark.

Cody, M., Beck, C., Courtney, R., & Shue, V. M. (2002). Integrating health services research into nursing doctoral programs: The evolution of nursing research. *Journal of Nursing Education, 41,* 207–214.

Cohen, M. A. (1998). Emerging trends in the finance and delivery of long-term care: Public and private opportunities and challenges. *Gerontologist, 38*(1), 80–89.

Cohen-Mansfield, J. (1997). Turnover among nursing home staff: A review. *Nursing Management, 28,* 59–62.

Cohen, J., Gorenberg, B., & Schroeder, B. (2000). A study of functional status among elders at two academic nursing centers. *Home Care Provider,* June, 108–112.

Cohen-Mansfield, J., Ejaz, F. K., & Werner, P. (Eds.) (2000). *Satisfaction surveys in long term care.* New York: Springer Publishing.

Cook, A. J. (1998). Cognitive-behavioral pain management for elderly nursing home residents. *Journal of Gerontology, 53B,* P51–P59.

Crown, W. H., Ahlburg, D. A., & MacAdam, M. (1995). The demographic and employment characteristics of home care aides: A comparison with nursing home aides, hospital aides, and other workers. *Gerontologist, 35,* 162–170.

Cubanski, J., & Kline, J. (April 2002). In Pursuit of Long Term Care: Ensuring Access, Coverage, Quality (Issue Brief). New York: The Commonwealth Fund.

Curry, L. (2002). Ethical and legal considerations in health services research. In M. B. Kapp, *Ethics, law, and aging review, Vol. 8: Issues in conducting research with and about older persons.* New York: Springer Publishing.

Dellasega, C., & Mastrian, K. (1995). The process and consequences of institutionalizing an elder. *Western Journal of Nursing Research, 17,* 123–136.

Dellefield, M. E. (2000). The relationship between nurse staffing in nursing homes and quality indicators: A literature review. *Journal of Gerontological Nursing, 26*(6), 15–28.

DeWolf Bosek, M. S., Savage, T. A., Anderson Shaw, L. A., & Renella, C. (2001). When surrogate decision-making is not straightforward: Guidelines for Nurse Administrators. *JONA's Law, Ethics, and Regulation, 3*(2), 47–55.

Diamond, J. (1999). *Guns, germs and steel: The fate of human societies.* New York: Norton.

Donabedian, A. (1966). Evaluating the quality of medical care. *Milbank Memorial Fund Quarterly, 44,* July (part 2), 166–203.

Dunbar, J. M., Neufeld, R. R., White, H. C., & Libow, L. S. (1996). Retrain, don't restrain: The educational intervention of the national nursing home restraint removal project. *Gerontologist, 36,* 539–542.

Eastman, P. (2002). More research needed on chronic conditions of the elderly. *Caring for the Aged, 3*(4), 1, 20, 22.

Eleazer, P., & Fretwell, M. (1999). The PACE model. In R. Katz, R. Kane, & M. Mezey (Eds.), *Emerging systems in long term care.* New York: Springer Publishing.

Elkan, R., Kendrick, D., Dewey, M., Hewitt, M., Robinson, J., Blair, M., Williams, D., & Brummell, K. (2001). Effectiveness of home based support for older people: Systematic review and meta-analysis. *British Medical Journal, 323,* 719–725.

Evans, J. M., Chutka, D. S., Fleming, K. C., Tangalos, E. G., Vittone, J., & Heathman, J. H. (1995). Medical care of nursing home residents. *Mayo Clinic Proceedings, 70,* 694–702.

Evans, L. K., Strumpf, N. E., Allen-Taylor, S. L., Capezuti, E., Maislin, G., & Jacobsen, B. (1997). A clinical trial to reduce restraints in nursing homes. *Journal of the American Geriatrics Society, 45,* 675–681.

Farrell-Miller, M. (1997). Physical aggressive resident behavior during hygiene care. *Journal of Gerontological Nursing, 23,* 24–39.

Feinsod, F. M., & Levenson, S. A. (1998). Procedures for managing ethical issues and medical decision making. *Annals of Long-Term Care, 6*(2), 63–65.

Feldman, P. H., Nadash, P., & Gursen, M. (2001). Improving communication between researchers and policy makers in long-term care: Or researchers are from Mars; Policy makers are from Venus. *The Gerontologist, 41*, 312–321.

Fink, S. V., & Picot, S. F. (1995). Nursing home placement decisions and post-placement experiences of African-American and European-American caregivers. *Journal of Gerontological Nursing, 21*, 35–42.

Fitch, S. M. (1990). Nursing Home as Neighborhood: A Systems Analysis of the American Nursing Home. Unpublished dissertation.

Fitzgerald, R. P., Shiverick, B. N., & Zimmerman, D. (1996). Applying performance measures to long-term care. *Joint Commission Journal on Quality Improvement, 22*(7), 505–517.

Folstein, M. F., Folstein, S. E., & Mc Hugh, P. R. (1975). Mini-mental state: A practical method for grading the cognitive state of patients for the clinician. *Journal of Psychiatric Research, 12*, 189–198.

Fonda, S. J., Clipp, E. C., & Maddox, G. L. (2002). Patterns in functioning among residents of an affordable assisted living housing facility. *The Gerontologist, 42*, 178–187.

Fost, N. (1997). When patients can't provide informed consent. *Chronicle of Higher Education, 48*(20), A48.

Friedemann, M. L., Montgomery, R. J., Rice, C., & Farrell, L. (1999). Family involvement in the nursing home. *Western Journal of Nursing Research, 21*, 549–567.

Fries, B. E. (1997). Changing the technology of assessing the elderly: The example of the R.A.I. *Generations,* Spring, 59–61.

Fries, B. E., Hawes, C., Morris, J. N., Phillips, C. D., Mor, V., & Park, P. S. (1997). Effect of the national resident assessment instrument on selected health conditions and problems. *Journal of the American Geriatrics Society, 45*, 994–1001.

Fries, B. E., Simon, S. E., Morris, J. N., Flodstrom, C., & Bookstein, F. L. (2001). Pain in U.S. nursing homes: Validating a pain scale for the minimum data set. *The Gerontologist, 41*, 173–179.

Fry, S. T., & Duffy, M. E. (2001). The development and psychometric evaluation of the ethical issues scale. *Journal of Nursing Scholarship, 33*(3), 273–277.

Frytak, J. R. (2001). Outcome trajectories for assisted living and nursing facility residents in Oregon. *Health Services Research, 36*, 91–111.

Gessert, C. E., Mosier, M. C., Brown, E. F., & Frey, B. (2000). Tube feeding in nursing home residents with severe and irreversible cognitive impairment. *Journal of the American Geriatrics Society, 48*, 1593–1600.

Giacolone, J. (2001). *The U. S. nursing home industry.* Armonk, NY: M. E. Sharpe.

Gloth, F. M., & Burton, J. R. (1990). Autopsies and death certificates in the chronic care setting. *Journal of the American Geriatrics Society, 38*, 151–155.

Gonzalez, A., & Marthon, F. G. (2000). Cultural diversity. *Advance for Nurses, 2*(3), 16–18.

Goodridge, D., & Hack, B. (1996). Assessing the congruence of nursing models with organizational culture: A quality improvement perspective. *Journal of Nursing Care Quality, 10*(2), 41–48.

Graber, D. R., & Sloane, P. D. (1995). Nursing home survey deficiencies for physical restraint use. *Medical Care, 33*, 1051–1063.

Grabowski, D. C. (2001). Medicaid reimbursement and the quality of nursing home care. *Journal of Health Economics, 20,* 549–569.

Grant, L. A., Kane, R. A., & Stark, A. J. (1995). Beyond labels: Nursing home care for Alzheimer's disease in and out of special care units. *Journal of the American Geriatrics Society, 43,* 569–576.

Grant, N. K., Reimer, M., & Bannatyne, J. (1996). Indicators of quality in long-term care facilities. *International Journal of Nursing Studies, 33,* 469–478.

Griffin, K. M. (1995). *Handbook of Sub-Acute Care.* Gaithersburg, MD: Aspen.

Gubrium, J. F. (1997). *Living and Dying at Murray Manor.* Charlottesville, VA: University of Virginia Press.

Gupta, S., Rappaport, H. M., & Bennett, L. T. (1996). Polypharmacy among nursing home geriatric Medicaid recipients. *Annals of Pharmacotherapy, 30,* 946–950.

Hale, B., Fong, V., & Dansky, K. (2001). Research says 'TeleHomecare' is cost effective, does not compromise care. *Legislative Network for Nurses, 18,* 165.

Hale, B., Fong, V., & Dansky, K. (2001). Advocates say staffing reduces use of chemical restraints in nursing homes. *Legislative Network for Nurses, 18,* 190.

Handy, J., Quinn, J., Ryan, M. A., & Wiener, J. (2002). Predictions—Long-term Care in the Decade. Available online: *http://www.nach.org/NAHC/NewsInfo/ni0600b.html.*

Hantikainen, V., & Kappeli, S. (2000). Using restraint with nursing home residents: A qualitative study of nursing staff perceptions and decision-making. *Journal of Advanced Nursing, 32,* 1196–1205.

Harrington, C., Carrillo, H., Thollaug, S. C., & Summers, P. R. (1997). Nursing Facilities, Staffing, Residents, and Facility Deficiencies, 1991 through 1995. Department of Social and Behavioral Sciences, University of California, San Francisco, CA.

Harrington, C., Mullan, J. M., Woodruff, L. C., Burger, S. G., Carillo, H., & Bedney, B. (1999). Stakeholders' opinions regarding important measures of nursing home quality for consumers. *Medical Care, 14,* 124–132.

Hartford Institute for Geriatric Nursing (1999). Staffing in nursing facilities. *Nursing Counts, 2*(2), 1–2.

Hawes, C., Morris, J. N., Phillips, C. D., Mor, V., Fries, B. E., & Nonemaker, S. (1995). Reliability estimates for the Minimum Data set (MDS) for nursing home resident assessment and care screening. *Gerontologist, 35,* 172–178.

Hawes, C., Mor, V., Phillips, C. D., Fries, B. E., Morris, J. N., Steele-Friedlob, E., Greene, A. M., & Nennstiel, M. (1997). The OBRA-87 nursing home regulations and implementation of the Resident Assessment Instrument: Effects on process quality. *Journal of the American Geriatrics Society, 45,* 977–985.

Hayley, D. C., Cassel, C. K., Snyder, L., & Rudberg, M. A. (1996). Ethical and legal issues in nursing home care. *Archives of Internal Medicine, 156,* 249–256.

Heath, H., McCormack, B., Phair, L., & Ford, P. (1996a). Developing outcome indicators in continuing care: Part 1. *Nursing Standard, 10*(46), 41–45.

Heath, H., McCormack, B., Phair, L., & Ford, P. (1996b). Developing outcome indicators in continuing care: Part 2. *Nursing Standard, 10*(47), 41–45.

Hershey, J. C., Collins, J. W., Gershon, R., & Owen, B. (1996). Methodologic issues in intervention research: Health care. *American Journal of Industrial Medicine, 29,* 412–417.

Hoffman, D. R. (1997). The federal effort to eliminate fraud and ensure quality care. *Advances in Wound Care, 10,* 36–38.

Holmes, J. S. (1996). The effects of ownership and ownership change on nursing home industry costs. *Health Services Research, 31,* 327–346.

Holtzman, J., & Lurie, N. (1996). Causes of increasing mortality in a nursing home population. *Journal of the American Geriatrics Society, 44,* 258–264.

Horowitz, A. (1997). The relationship between vision impairment and the assessment of disruptive behaviors among nursing home residents. *Gerontologist, 37,* 620–628.

Hudson, K. A., & Sexton, D. L. (1996). Perceptions about nursing care: Comparing elders' and nurses' priorities. *Journal of Gerontological Nursing, 22*(12), 41–46.

Hughes, S. L., Ulasevich, A., Weaver, F. M., Henderson, W., Manheim, L., Kubal, J. D., & Bonargio, F. (1997). Impact of home care on hospital days: A meta-analysis. *Health Services Research, 32,* 415–432.

Ignatavicius, D. D. (1998). *Introduction to long term care nursing: Principles and practices.* Philadelphia: F. A. Davis.

Institute for Health and Aging, University of California, San Francisco (1996). *Chronic care in America: A 21st century challenge.* Princeton, NJ: Robert Wood Johnson Foundation.

Jackson, M. E., Spector, W. D., & Rabins, P. V. (1997). Risk of behavior problems among nursing home residents in the United States. *Journal of Aging and Health, 9*(4), 451–472.

Jaffe, M. (1999). *Geriatric long-term procedures and treatments,* 2nd ed. Englewood, CO: Skidmore-Roth Publishing.

Jaffe, M. (1998). *The OBRA guidelines for quality improvement,* 3rd ed., rev. Englewood, CO: Skidmore-Roth Publishing.

Jirovec, M. M., & Templin, T. (2001). Predicting success using individualized scheduled toileting for memory-impaired elders at home. *Research in Nursing and Health, 24*(1), 1–8.

Johnson, B. D., Stone, G. L., Altmaier, E. M., & Berdahl, L. D. (1998). The relationship of demographic factors, locus of control and self-efficacy to successful nursing home adjustment. *Gerontologist, 38,* 209–216.

Johnston, D., & Reifler, B. V. (1999). Comprehensive Care for Older People with Alzheimer's Disease. In E. Calkins, C. Boult, E. H. Wagner, & J. T. Pacala (Eds.), *New ways to care for older people: Building systems based on evidence.* New York: Springer Publishing.

Kane, R. A. (1995a). Ethical themes in long term care. In P. R. Katz, R. L. Kane, & M. D. Mezey (Eds.), *Quality care in geriatric settings.* New York: Springer Publishing.

Kane, R. L. (1995b). Improving the quality of long-term care. *Journal of the American Medical Association, 273,* 1376–1380.

Kane, R. L. (1996). The evolution of the American nursing home. In R. H. Binstock, L. E. Cluff, & O. von Mering (Eds.), *The future of long-term care: Social and policy issues.* Baltimore: Johns Hopkins University Press.

Kane, R. A. (2001). Long-term care and a good quality of life: Bringing them closer together. *The Gerontologist, 41*(3), 293–304.

Kane, R. L., Chen, Q., Blewitt, L. A., & Sangl, J. (1996). Do rehabilitative nursing homes improve the outcomes of care? *Journal of the American Geriatrics Society, 44,* 545–554.

Kane, R. L., & Kane, R. A. (1995). Long-term care. *Journal of the American Medical Association, 273*(21), 1690–1691.

Kane, R. L., & Kane, R. A. (2001). What older people want from long-term care, and how they can get it. *Health Affairs, 20*(6), 114–127.

Kane, R. A., Kane, R. L., & Ladd, R. C. (1998). *The heart of long term care.* New York: Oxford University Press.

Kapp, M. B. (1994). *Patient self-determination in long term care.* New York: Springer Publishing.

Kapp, M. B. (2000). Testing consumer-directed models of long-term care: Ethical and legal considerations. In M. B. Kapp, *Ethics, law, and aging, vol. 6: Consumer-directed care and the older person.* New York: Springer Publishing.

Kari, N., & Michels, P. (1991). The Lazarus project: The politics of empowerment. *American Journal of Occupational Therapy, 45,* 719–725.

Karon, S. L., & Zimmerman, D. R. (1998). Nursing home quality indicators and quality improvement initiatives. *Top Health Information Management, 18*(4), 46–58.

Karon, S. L., Sainfort, F., & Zimmerman, D. R. (1999). Stability of nursing home indicators over time. *Medical Care, 37,* 570–579.

Kartes, S. K. (1996). A team approach for risk assessment, prevention, and treatment of pressure ulcers in nursing home patients. *Journal of Nursing Care Quality, 10*(3), 34–45.

Katz, S., Ford, A. B., Moskowitz, R. W., Jackson, B. A., & Jaffe, M. W. (1963). The index of ADL: A standardized measure of biological and psychosocial function. *Journal of the American Medical Association, 185,* 914–919.

Katz, P. R., Kane, R. L., & Mezey, M. D. (Eds.). (1999). *Emerging systems in long-term care.* New York: Springer Publishing.

Kingston, P., Bernard, M., Biggs, S., & Nettleton, H. (2001). Assessing the health impact of age-specific housing. *Health and Social Care in the Community, 9,* 228–234.

Kjervik, D. K., Weisensee, M. G., Anderson, J., & Carlson, J. R. (1998). A comparison of assessments made by nurses, informal caregivers, and legal professionals of incapacity criteria for guardianship of older persons. *American Journal of Alzheimer's Disease, 13*(1), 34–39.

Klauber, K. (2000). Eden a place to live. *Advance for Nurses, 2*(3), 14–15.

Koroknay, V. J., Werner, P., Cohen-Mansfield, J., & Braun, J. V. (1995). Maintaining ambulation in the frail nursing home resident: A nursing administered walking program. *Journal of Gerontological Nursing, 21,* 18–24.

Kovach, C. R., & Krejci, J. W. (1998). Facilitating change in dementia care. *Journal of Nursing Administration, 28*(5), 17–27.

Kovner, C., & Harrington, C. (2001). Strengthening the caregiving workforce. *American Journal of Nursing, 101*(9), 55–56.

Kovner, C., & Harrington, C. (2002). Nursing care providers in home care: A shortage of nonprofessional, direct care staff. *American Journal of Nursing, 102*(1), 91–92.

Kovner, C., & Harrington, C. (2003). Nursing care in assisted living facilities. *American Journal of Nursing, 103*(1), 97–98.

Krauss, N. A., Freiman, M. P., Rhoades, J. A., Altman, B. M., Brown Jr., E., & Potter, D. E. (1997). Agency for Health Care Policy and Research, Nursing Home Update, 1996 Medical Expenditure Panel Survey. *Highlights,* July, Number 2.

Kruzich, J. M. (1995). Empowering organizational contexts: Patterns and predictors of perceived decision-making influence among staff in nursing homes. *Gerontologist, 35*, 207–216.

Kunin, C. M., Douthitt, S., Dancing, J., Anderson, J., & Moeschlberger, M. (1992). The association between the use of urinary catheters and morbidity and mortality among elderly patients in nursing homes. *American Journal of Epidemiology, 135*, 291–301.

Kurlander, S. S., & Scherb, E. (1997). Liability under the False Claims Act for inadequate care of nursing facility residents. *Advances in Wound Care, 10*, 47–49.

Landi, F., Onder, G., Tua, E., Carrara, B., Gambassi, G., Carbonin, P., & Bernabei, R. (2001). Impact of a new assessment system, the MDS-HC, on function and hospitalization of homebound older people: A controlled clinical trial. *Journal of the American Geriatrics Society, 49*, 1299–1293.

Lang, J. M. (1990). The use of a run-in to enhance compliance. *Stat Med, 9*, 87–95.

Langer, E., Drinka, P. J., & Voeks, S. (1991). Readmission and acuity in the nursing home: How will the nursing homes manage? *Journal of Gerontological Nursing, 17*, 15–19.

Lawrence, F. C., Moser, E. B., Prawitz, A. D., & Collier, M. W. (1995). Gender differences in the financing of nursing home care. *Psychological Reports, 77*, 1169–1170.

Lawton, M. P. (1975). The Philadelphia Geriatric Morale Scale: A revision. *Journal of Gerontology, 30*, 85–89.

Lekan-Rutledge, D. (2000). Diffusion of innovation: A model of prompted voiding in long-term care settings. *Journal of Gerontological Nursing, 26*(4), 25–33.

Lemke, S., & Moos, R. H. (1987). Measuring the social climate of congregate residences for older people: The sheltered care environment scale. *Psychology of Aging, 2*, 20–29.

Li, J., Birkhead, G. S., Strogatz, D. S., & Coles, F. B. (1996). Impact of institution size, staffing patterns, and infection control practices on communicable disease outbreaks in New York State nursing homes. *American Journal of Epidemiology, 143*, 1042–1049.

Lieberman, T., & the Editors of Consumer Reports (2000). *Consumer reports complete guide to health services for seniors.* New York: Three Rivers Press.

Lindrooth, R. C., Hoerger, T. J., & Norton, E. C. (2000). Expectations among the elderly about nursing home entry. *Health Services Research, 35*(5), 1181–1202.

Lipowski, E. E., & Bigelow, W. E. (1996). Data linkages for research on outcomes of long term care. *Gerontologist, 36*, 441–447.

Lipsitz, L. A., Pluchino, F. C., & Wright, S. M. (1987). Biomedical research in the nursing home: Methodological issues and subject recruitment results. *Journal of the American Geriatrics Society, 35*, 629–634.

Loeb, J. L. (1999). Pain management in long-term care. *American Journal of Nursing, 99*, 48–52.

Loeb, M., Moss, L., Stiller, A., Smith, S., Russo, R., & Molloy, D. W. (2001). Colonization with multiresistant bacteria and quality of life of residents in long-term care. *Infection Control and Hospital Epidemiology, 22*(2), 67–68.

Lohr, K. N., & Steinwachs, D. M. (2002). Health services research: An evolving definition of the field. *Health Services Research, 37*, 7–9.

Long Term Care Education.com. (2002). Definition of the types of residential care. Available online: *http://www.longtermcareeducation.com/A1/a.asp*: Author.

Long Term Care Education.com. (2002). Definition of assisted living. Available online: *http://www.longtermcareeducation.com/A1/a.asp*: Author.

Long Term Care Education.com. (2002). Get an overview of the long term care industry today. Available online: *http://www.longtermcareeducation.com/A1/a.asp*: Author.

Loue, S. (2002). Ethical issues in informed consent in the conduct of research with aging persons. In M. B. Kapp, *Ethics, law, and aging review, vol. 8: Issues in conducting research with and about older persons.* New York: Springer Publishing.

Lynn, J. (1992). Procedures for making decisions for incompetent adults. *Journal of the American Medical Association, 267,* 2082–2084.

Lyons. S. S., & Pringle-Specht, J. K. (2000). Prompted voiding protocol for individuals with urinary incontinence. *Journal of Gerontological Nursing, 26*(6), 5–13.

McBride. A. B. (2000). Nursing and gerontology. *Journal of Gerontological Nursing, 26*(7), 18–27.

McCann, R. M., Hall, W. J., & Groth-Juncker, A. (1994). Comfort care for terminally ill patients: The appropriate use of nutrition and hydration. *Journal of the American Medical Association, 272,* 1263–1266.

McCann, R. M. (1999). Care of older people who are dying. In E. Calkins, C. Boult, E. H. Wagner, & J. T. Pacala (Eds.), *New ways to care for older people: Building systems based on evidence.* New York: Springer Publishing.

McCullough, L. B., & Wilson, N. L. (1995). *Long-term care decisions: Ethical and conceptual dimensions.* Baltimore: Johns Hopkins University Press.

McDougall, G. J. (1990). A review of screening instruments for assessing cognition and mental status in older adults. *Nurse Practitioner, 15,* 18–28.

McHorney, C. A. (1996). Measuring and monitoring general health status in elderly persons: Practical and methodological issues in using the SF-36 health survey. *Gerontologist, 36,* 571–583.

MacRae, P. G., Asplund, L. A., Schnelle, J. F., Ouslander, J. G., Abrahamse, A., & Morris, C. (1996). A walking program for nursing home residents: Effects on walk endurance, physical activity, mobility, and quality of life. *Journal of the American Geriatrics Society, 44,* 175–180.

Magaziner, J., German, P., Zimmerman, S. I., Hebel, R., Burton, L., Gruber-Baldini, A. L., May, C., & Kittner, S. (2000). *The Gerontologist, 40,* 663–672.

Marek, D. K., Rantz, M. J., Fagin, C. M., & Wessel Krejci, J. (1996a). OBRA '87: Has it resulted in better quality of care? *Journal of Gerontological Nursing,* October, 28–35.

Marek, D. K., Rantz, M. J., Fagin, C. M., & Wessel Krejci, J. (1996b). OBRA '87: Has it resulted in positive change in nursing homes? *Journal of Gerontological Nursing,* December, 32–39.

Mark, D. H., Bahr, J., Duthie, E. H., & Tresch, D. D. (1995). Characteristics of residents with do-not-resuscitate orders. *Archives of Family Medicine, 4,* 463–467.

Mathieson, K. M., Kronenfeld, J. J., & Keith, V. M. (2002). Maintaining functional independence in elderly adults: The roles of health status and financial resources in predicting home modifications and use of mobility equipment. *The Gerontologist, 42,* 24–31.

Matteson, M. A., Linton, A. D., Cleary, B. L., Barnes, S. J., & Lichtenstein, M. J. (1997). Management of problematic behavioral symptoms associated with dementia: A cognitive developmental approach. *Aging: Clinical and Experimental Research, 9,* 342–355.

Mattiasson, A. C., & Andersson, L. (1994). Staff attitude and experience in dealing with rational nursing home patients who refuse to eat and drink. *Journal of Advanced Nursing, 20,* 822–827.

Mattiasson, A. C., & Andersson, L. (1995). Organizational environment and the support of patient autonomy in nursing home care. *Journal of Advanced Nursing, 22,* 1149–1157.

Mehr, D. R., & Fries, B. E. (1995). Resource use on Alzheimer's special care units. *Gerontologist, 35,* 179–184.

Meredith, S., Feldman, P. H., Frey, D., Hall, K., Arnold, K., Brown, N. J., & Ray, W. A. (2001). Possible medication errors in home healthcare patients. *Journal of the American Geriatrics Society, 49,* 719–724.

Mezey, M. D., Mitty, E. L., & Bottrel, M. (1997). The teaching nursing home program: Enduring educational outcomes. *Nursing Outlook, 45*(3), 133–140.

Mezey, M., Mitty, E., & Ramsey, G. (1997). Assessment of decision-making capacity: Nursing's role. *Journal of Gerontological Nursing, 23*(3), 28–35.

Miller, S., Gozalo, P., & Mor, V. (2001). Hospice enrollment and hospitalization of dying nursing home patients. *American Journal of Medicine, 111,* 38–44.

Miller, D. K., Coe, R. M., Morley, J. E., & Romeis, J. C. (1995). *Total quality management in geriatric care.* New York: Springer Publishing.

Mohs, R. C. (1987). Alzheimer's disease: Morbid risk among first-degree relatives approximates 50% by 90 years of age. *Archives of General Psychiatry, 44,* 405–408.

Moos, R. H., & Lemke, S. (1984). Multiphasic Environmental Assessment Procedure (MEAP) Manual. Sheltered Care Project, Social Ecology Laboratory and Geriatric Research, Education and Clinical Center, Veterans Administration and Stanford University Medical Center, Palo Alto, CA.

Mor, V. (1995). Invest in your frontline worker: Commentary. *Brown University Long-term Care Quality Letter, 7*(1), 4–5.

Mor, V., Branco, K., Fleishman, J., Hawes, C., Phillips, C., Morris, J., & Fries, B. (1995). The structure of social engagement for nursing home residents. *Journals of Gerontology, 50B,* P1–P8.

Mor, V., Intrator, O., Fries, B. E., Phillips, C., Teno, J., Hiris, J., Hawes, C., & Morris, J. (1997). Changes in hospitalization associated with introducing the resident assessment instrument. *Journal of the American Geriatrics Society, 45,* 1002–1010.

Morgan, D. G., Semchuk, K. M., Stewart, N. J., & D'Arcy, C. (2002). Job strain among staff of rural nursing homes. *The Journal of Nursing Administration, 32,* 152–161.

Morris, J. N., Lipsitz, L. A., Murphy, K., & Bellville-Taylor, P. (1997b). *Quality care in the nursing home.* St. Louis: Mosby Lifeline.

Morris, J. N., Nonemaker, S., Murphy, K., Hawes, C., Fries, B. E., Mor, V., & Phillips, C. (1997a). A commitment to change: Revision of HCFA's R.A.I. *Journal of the American Geriatrics Society, 45,* 1011–1016.

Morrow-Howell, N., Proctor, E., & Rozario, P. (2001). How much is enough? Perspectives of care recipients and professionals on the sufficiency of in-home care. *Gerontologist, 41*(6), 723–732.

Mueller, C., & Cam, H. (2002). Comprehensive management of urinary incontinence through quality improvement efforts. *Geriatric Nursing, 23,* 82–87.

Mueller, C. (2000). The RUG-III case mix classification system for long-term care nursing facilities: Is it adequate for nursing staff? *Journal of Nursing Administration, 30*(11), 535–543.

Mukamel, D. B. (1997). Risk-adjusted outcome measures and quality of care in nursing homes. *Medical Care, 35*, 367–385.

Murphy, K. M., Morris, J. N., Fries, B. E., & Zimmerman, D. R. (1995–1996). The Resident Assessment Instrument: Implications for quality, reimbursement, and research. *Generations*, Winter, 43–46.

Murtaugh, C. M., Kemper, P., Spillman, B. C., & Carson, B. L. (1997). The amount, distribution, and timing of lifetime nursing home use. *Medical Care, 35*(3), 204–218.

National Academy on Aging (1997). *Facts on long-term care*. Washington, DC: Author.

National Association for Home Care (2002). What is Hospice? Available online: *http://www.nahc.org/NACH/NewsInfo/hospice.html*.

National Association for Home Care (2002). What services are provided by home care agencies? Available online: *http://www.nahc.org/NAHC/NewsInfo/svcs_homecare.html*.

National Committee to Preserve Social Security and Medicare (2000). Legislative agenda for the 106th Congress: Nurse staffing in nursing homes. Washington, DC: Author.

National Institutes of Health (1998, February). Research involving individuals with questionable capacity to consent: Ethical and practical considerations for institutional review boards. Expert Panel Report. Washington, DC: Author.

Naylor, M. D., & Prior, P. R. (1999). Transitions between acute and long term care. In P. R. Katz, R. L. Kane, & M. D. Mezey (Eds.), *Emerging systems in long-term care*. New York: Springer Publishing.

Nicolle, L. E., Bentley, D., Garibaldi, R., Neuhaus, E., & Smith, P. (1996). Antimicrobial use in long-term-care facilities. *Infection Control and Hospital Epidemiology, 17*, 119–128.

Noel, H. C., & Vogel, D. C. (2000). Resource costs and quality of life outcomes for homebound elderly using telemedicine integrated with nurse case management. *Care Management, 6*(5), 22–24, 26–28, 30–31.

North Carolina Assisted Living Association (2002). Who is the North Carolina assisted living association? *NC Assisted Living News*, March, 6.

Office of the Inspector General (2001). Psychotropic drug use in nursing homes: Supplemental information. Available online: *http://oig.hhs.gov/oei/reports/oei-02-00-00490.pdf*.

Ooi, W. L., Sherwood, S., Murphy, K., Morris, S. A., & Morris, J. N. (1996). Development, testing, and validation of two scales measuring nursing home management of subjects with mental disorder. *Journal of Clinical Epidemiology, 49*, 1381–1388.

Opus Communications (2000). *Continuous quality improvement for long-term care*. Marblehead, MA: Author.

Ouslander, J. G., & Schnelle, J. F. (1993). Research in nursing homes: Practical aspects. *Journal of the American Geriatrics Society, 41*, 182–187.

Ouslander, J. D., Schnelle, J. F., Uman, G., Fingold, S., Nigam, J. G., Tuico, E., & Bates-Jensen, B. (1995). Predictors of successful prompted voiding among incontinent nursing home residents. *Journal of the American Medical Association, 273*, 1366–1370.

Patterson, B. J. (1994). Reflections of a nurse researcher in a nursing home. *Geriatric Nursing, 15*, 198–200.

Phillips, C. D., Hawes, C., Mor, V., Fries, B. E., Morris, J. N., & Nennstiel, M. E. (1996). Facility and area variation affecting the use of physical restraints in nursing homes. *Medical Care, 34*, 1139–1162.

Phillips, C. D., Morris, J. N., Hawes, C., Fries, B. E., Mor, V., Nennstiel, M. E., & Iannacchione, V. (1997). Association of the resident assessment instrument with changes in function, cognition, and psychosocial status. *Journal of the American Geriatrics Society, 45,* 986–993.

Phillips, C. (2002). Yali's question and the study of nursing homes as organizations. *The Gerontologist, 42*(2), 154–156.

Phillips, L. R., & Van Ort, S. (1995). Issues in conducting intervention research in long-term care settings. *Nursing Outlook, 43,* 249–253.

Plutchnik, R., Conte, H., Liegerman, M., Bakur, M., Grossman, J., & Lehman, N. (1970). Reliability and validity of a scale for assessing the functioning of geriatric patients. *Journal of the American Geriatrics Society, 18,* 491–500.

Powers, B. A. (2001). Ethnographic analysis of everyday ethics in the care of nursing home residents with dementia. *Nursing Research, 50,* 332–339.

Proenca, E. J., & Shewchuk, R. M. (1997). Organizational tenure and the perceived importance of retention factors in nursing homes. *Health Care Management Review, 22,* 65–73.

Pruchno, R. A., Smyer, M. A., Rose, M. S., Hartman-Stein, P. E., & Henderson-Laribee (1995). Competence of long-term care residents to participate in decisions about their medical care: A brief, objective assessment. *The Gerontologist, 35,* 622–629.

Przybylski, B. R., Dumont, E. D., Watkins, M. E., Warren, S. A., Beaulne, A. P., & Lier, D. A. (1996). Outcomes of enhanced physical and occupational therapy service in a nursing home setting. *Archives of Physical Medicine and Rehabilitation, 77,* 554–561.

Ramsay, J. D., Sainfort, F., & Zimmerman, D. (1995). An empirical test of the structure, process, and outcome quality paradigm using resident-based, nursing facility assessment data. *American Journal of Medical Quality, 10*(2), 63–75.

Rantz, M. J., Vinz-Miller, T., & Matson, S. (1995). Nursing diagnosis in long-term care: A longitudinal perspective for strategic planning. *Nursing Diagnosis, 6,* 57–63.

Rantz, M. J., Mehr, D. R., Conn, V. S., Hicks, L. L., Porter, R., Madsen, R. W., Petrowski, G. F., & Maas, M. (1996). Assessing quality of nursing home care: The foundation for improving resident outcomes. *Journal of Nursing Care Quality, 10,* 1–9.

Rantz, M. J., & Popejoy, L. L. (1998). *Using MDS quality indicators to improve outcomes.* Gaithersburg, MD: Aspen Publishers, Inc.

Rantz, M. J., Popejoy, L., Mehr, D. R., Zwygart-Stauffacher, M., Hicks, L. L., Grando, V., Conn, V., Porter, R., Scott, J., & Maas, M. (1997). Verifying nursing home care quality using minimum data set quality indicators and other quality measures. *Journal of Nursing Care Quality, 12*(2), 54–62.

Rantz, M. J., Popejoy, L., Zwygart-Stauffacher, M., Wipke Tevis, D., & Grando, V. (1999). Minimum Data Set and Resident Assessment Instrument: Can using standardized assessment improve clinical practice and outcomes of care? *Journal of Gerontological Nursing, 25*(6), 35–43.

Rantz, M. J., Zwygart-Stauffacher, M., Popejoy, L., Grando, V., Mehr, D. R., Hicks, L. L., Conn, V., & Wipke Tevis, D. (1999). Nursing home care quality: A multidimensional theoretical model integrating the views of consumers and providers. *Journal of Nursing Care Quality, 14*(1), 16–37.

Rantz, M. J., Mehr, D. R., Petroski, G., Madsen, R., Popejoy, L., Hicks, L. L., Conn, V., Grando, V., Wipke Tevis, D., Bostick, J., Porter, R., Zwygart-Stauffacher, M., & Maas,

M. (2000). Initial field testing of an instrument to measure observable indicators of nursing home care quality. *Journal of Nursing Care Quality, 15*(3), 1–12.

Rantz, M. J., Marek, K., & Zwygart-Stauffacher, M. (2000). The future of long term care for the chronically ill. *Nursing Administration Quarterly, 25*(1), 51–58.

Rantz, M. J., Popejoy, L., Petroski, G., Madsen, R., Mehr, D. R., Zwygart-Stauffacher, M., Hicks, L. L., Grando, V., WipkeTevis, D., Bostick, J., Porter, R., Conn, V., & Maas, M. (2001). Randomized clinical trial of a quality improvement intervention in nursing homes. *The Gerontologist, 41*, 525–538.

Rapp, C. G., Topps-Uriri, J., & Beck, C. (1994). Obtaining and maintaining a research sample with cognitively impaired nursing home residents. *Geriatric Nursing, 15*, 193–196.

Ray, W. A., Taylor, J. A., Meador, K. G., Thapa, P. B., Brown, A. K., Kajihara, H. K., Davis, C., Gideon, P., & Griffin, M. R. (1997). A randomized trial of a consultation service to reduce falls in nursing homes. *Journal of the American Medical Association, 278*, 557–562.

Reinhard, S., & Stone, R. (2001). *Promoting quality in nursing homes: The Wellspring Model.* New York: The Commonwealth Fund.

Reschovsky, J. D. (1996). Demand for and access to institutional long-term care: The role of Medicaid in nursing home markets. *Inquiry, 33*, 15–29.

Resnick, B. (1999). Falls in a community of older adults: Putting research into practice. *Clinical Nursing Research, 8*, 251–266.

Resnick, B. (2001). The restoration of independence. *American Journal of Nursing, 101*(10), 11.

Resnick, H. E., Fries, B. E., & Verbrugge, L. M. (1997). Windows to their world: The effect of sensory impairments on social engagement and activity time in nursing home residents. *Journal of Gerontology, 52B*, S135–44.

Rhoades, J. A., & Krauss, N. A. (1999). Nursing Home Trends, 1987 and 1996 (MEPS Chartbook #3), Publication Number 99-0032. Rockville, MD: Agency for Healthcare Research and Quality.

Robertson, J. F., & Cummings, C. C. (1996). Attracting nurses to long-term care. *Journal of Gerontological Nursing, 22*(9), 24–32.

Rosen, C. S., Chow, H. C., Greenbaum, M. A., Finney, J. F., Moos, R. F., Sheikh, J. I., & Yesavage, J. A. (2002). How well are clinicians following dementia practice guidelines? *Alzheimer Disease and Related Disorders, 16*(1), 15–23.

Rosko, M. D., Chilingerian, J. A., Zinn, J. S., & Aaronson, W. E. (1995). The effects of ownership, operating environment, and strategic choices on nursing home efficiency. *Medical Care, 33*, 1001–1021.

Ross, M. M., & Crook, J. (1998). Elderly recipients of nursing home services: Pain, disability, and functional competence. *Journal of Advanced Nursing, 27*, 1117–1126.

Roubenoff, R., Giacoppe, J., Richardson, S., & Hoffman, P. J. (1996). Nutrition assessment in long-term care facilities. *Nutrition Reviews, 54*(1 Pt 2), S40–2.

Rowles, G. D., Beaulieu, J. E., & Myers, W. W. (1996). *Long-term care for the rural elderly: New directions in services, research, and policy.* New York: Springer Publishing.

Russo, H. E. (2002). Home care in the 21st century. Available online: *http://www.nahc.org/NAHC/NewsInfo/ni1101.html.*

Ryden, M. B., Snyder, M., Gross, C. R., Savik, K., Pearson, V., Krichbaum, K., & Mueller, C. (2000). Value-added outcomes: The use of advanced practice nurses in long-term care facilities. *The Gerontologist, 40*(6), 654–662.

Sachs, G. A., Rhymes, J., & Cassel, C. K. (1993). Biomedical and behavioral research in nursing homes: Guidelines for ethical investigations. *Journal of the American Geriatrics Society, 41,* 771–777.

Sainfort, F., Ramsay, J. D., Ferreira, P. L., & Mezghani, L. (1994). A first step in total quality management of nursing facility care: Development of an empirical causal model of structure, process and outcome dimensions. *American Journal of Medical Quality, 9*(2), 74–86.

Schnelle, J. F., Cruise, P. A., Alessi, C. A., Al-Samarrai, N., & Ouslander, J. G. (1998). Individualizing nighttime incontinence care in nursing home residents. *Nursing Research, 47*(4), 197–203.

Schnelle, J. F., McNees, P., Crooks, V., & Ouslander, J. G. (1995). The use of a computer-based model to implement an incontinence management program. *Gerontologist, 35,* 656–665.

Schnelle, J. F., Ouslander, J. G., Buchanan, J., Zellman, G., Farley, D., Hirsch, S. H., & Reuben, D. B. (1999). Objective and subjective measures of the quality of managed care in nursing homes. *Medical Care, 37,* 375–383.

Schnelle, J. F., & Reuben, D. B. (1999). Long-term care in the nursing home. In E. Calkins, C. Boult, E. H. Wagner, & J. T. Pacala (Eds.), *New ways to care for older people: Building systems based on evidence.* New York: Springer Publishing.

Schwarz, K. A. (2000). Predictors of early hospital admissions for older adults who are functionally impaired. *Journal of Gerontological Nursing, 26*(6), 29–36.

Shelton, B. (2002). HIPAA wires healthcare: Will assisted living be part of the circuit? *NC Assisted Living News, 1*(3), 8–9.

Silberman, P. C., Weisner, K. K., Leysieffer, K. E., Freund, C. M., Bruton, H. D., Ingram, R. A., & DeFriese, G. H. (2002). A long-term care plan for North Carolina: Synopsis of the North Carolina Institute of Medicine final report. *North Carolina Medical Journal, 63,* 80–82.

Simmons, S. F., Schnelle, J. F., Uman, G. C., Kulvicki, A. D., Lee, K. H., & Ouslander, J. G. (1997). Selecting nursing home residents for satisfaction surveys. *Gerontologist, 37,* 543–550.

Simmons, S. F., & Schnelle, J. F. (1999). Strategies to measure nursing home residents' satisfaction and preferences related to incontinence and mobility care: Implications for evaluating intervention effects. *Gerontologist, 39,* 345–355.

Slaets, J. P., Kauffmann, R. H., Duivenvoorden, H. J., Pelemans, W., & Schudel, W. J. (1997). A randomized trial of geriatric liaison intervention in elderly medical inpatients. *Psychosomatic Medicine, 59,* 585–591.

Sloane, P. D., Lindeman, D. A., Phillips, C., Moritz, D. J., & Koch, G. (1995). Evaluating Alzheimer's special care units: Reviewing the evidence and identifying potential sources of study bias. *Gerontologist, 35,* 103–111.

Smith, G. P. (1996). *Legal and healthcare ethics for the elderly.* Washington, DC: Taylor and Francis.

Smyer, M., Schaie, K. W., & Kapp, M. B. (1996). *Older adults' decision-making and the law.* New York: Springer Publishing.

Sorlie, T., Sexton, H. C., Busund, R., & Sorlie, D. (2001). A Global measure of physical functioning: Psychometric properties. *Health Services Research, 36,* 1109–1124.

Spector, W. D., & Fleishman, J. A. (1998). Combining activities of daily living with instrumental activities of daily living to measure functional disability. *Journal of Gerontology: Social Sciences, 53,* S46–S57.

Spector, W. D., Reschovsky, J. D., & Cohen, J. W. (1996). Appropriate placement of nursing-home residents in lower levels of care. *Milbank Quarterly, 74,* 139–160.

Spore, D. L., Mor, V., Larrat, P., Hawes, C., & Hiris, J. (1997). Inappropriate drug prescriptions for elderly residents of board and care facilities. *American Journal of Public Health, 87,* 404–409.

Sprung, C., & Eidelman, L. (1996). Judicial intervention in medical decision-making: A failure of the medical system? *Critical Care Medicine, 24*(5), 730–732.

Stackhouse, J. C. (1998). *Into the community: Nursing in ambulatory and home care.* Philadelphia: Lippincott.

Stanhope, M., & Knollmueller, R. N. (2000). *Handbook of community-based home health and nursing practice.* St. Louis: Mosby.

Steffen, T. M., & Mollinger, L. A. (1995). Low-load, prolonged stretch in the treatment of knee flexion contractures in nursing home residents. *Physical Therapy, 75,* 886–895.

Stein, W. M., & Ferrell, B. A. (1996). Pain in the nursing home. *Clinics in Geriatric Medicine, 12,* 601–613.

Stevens, J. A., & Olson, S. (2000). Reducing falls and resulting hip fractures among older women. *Home Care Provider,* August, 134–139.

Stevenson, K. B. (1999). Regional data set of infection rates of long-term care facilities: Description of a valuable benchmarking tool. *American Journal of Infection Control, 27,* 20–26.

Sullivan, E. J. (2002). Top 10 reasons a manuscript is rejected. *Journal of Professional Nursing, 18,* 1–2.

Sumaya-Smith, I. (1995). Caregiver/resident relationships: Surrogate family bonds and surrogate grieving in a skilled nursing facility. *Journal of Advanced Nursing, 21,* 447–451.

Suri, D. N., Egleston, B. L., Brody, J. A., & Rudberg, M. A. (1999). Nursing home resident use of care directives. *Journals of Gerontology, Series A: Biological and Medical Sciences, 54,* M225–229.

Teno, J. M., Licks, S., Lynn, J., Wenger, N., Connors, A. F., Phillips, R. S., O'Connor, M. A., Murphy, D. P., Fulkerson, W. J., Desbiens, N., & Knaus, W. A. (1997a). Do advance directive provide instructions that direct care? *Journal of the American Geriatrics Society, 45,* 508–512.

Teno, J. M., Branco, K. J., Mor, V., Phillips, C. D., Hawes, C., Morris, J., & Fries, B. E. (1997b). Changes in advance care planning in nursing homes before and after the patient self-determination act: Report of a 10-state survey. *Journal of the American Geriatrics Society, 45,* 939–944.

Teno, J. M. (2002). Now is the time to embrace nursing homes as a place of care for dying persons. *Innovations in End-of-Life Care, 4*(2). Available online: *http://www2.edc.org/lastacts/editorial.asp*

Thomas, S., Senior Vice-President of NC Association for Home and Hospice Care (2003). Personal communication, February 4.

Thomas, W. H. (1996). *A life worth living.* Acton, MA: Vanderwyk and Burnham.

Tinetti, M. E., Doucette, J. T., & Claus, E. B. (1995). The contribution of predisposing and situational risk factors to serious fall injuries. *Journal of the American Gerontological Society, 43,* 1207–1213.

Toye, C., Percival, P., & Blackmore, A. (1996). Satisfaction with nursing home care of a relative: Does inviting greater input make a difference? *Collegian, 3,* 4–11.

U.S. General Accounting Office (1997). Long-term care: Consumer protection and quality of care issues in assisted living. Washington, DC: Author. ·

Vap, P. W., & Dunaye, T. (2000). Pressure ulcer risk assessment in long-term care nursing. *Journal of Gerontological Nursing, 26*(6), 37–45.

Voelkl, J. E., Galecki, A. T., & Fries, B. E. (1996). Nursing home residents with severe cognitive impairments: Predictors of participation in activity groups. *Therapeutic Recreation Journal,* First quarter, 27–40.

Wallace, S. P., Levy-Storms, L., Kington, R. S., & Andersen, R. M. (1998). The persistence of race and ethnicity in the use of long-term care. *Journal of Gerontology: Social Sciences, 53B*(2), S104–12.

Walshe, K. (2001). Regulating U.S. nursing homes: Are we learning from experience? *Health Affairs, 20*(6), 128–144.

Watson, N. W. (2002). Application of the AHCPR urinary incontinence guideline in nursing homes. *AHRQ Research Activities, 267,* December, 2002, 15.

Watt, H. M. (2001). Community-based case management: A model for outcome-based research for non-institutionalized elderly. *Home Health Care Services Quarterly, 20*(1), 39–59.

Weinberg, A. D., & Minaker, K. L. (1995). Dehydration: Evaluation and management in older adults. *Journal of the American Medical Association, 274,* 1552–1556.

Weisenssee, M. G., & Kjervik, D. (2001). Assessment of cognitively impaired elderly: A challenge for public policy in an aging society. *Journal of Nursing Law, 8*(1), 33–47.

Weissert, W. W., & Hedrick, S. C. (1999). Outcomes and costs of home and community-based long-term care: Implications for research-based practice. In E. Calkins, C. Boult, E. H. Wagner, & J. T. Pacala, *New ways to care for older people: Building systems based on evidence.* New York: Springer Publishing.

White, G. (2001). *Code of Ethics for Nurses, 101*(10), 73, 75.

Wicclair, M. R. (1993). *Ethics and the Elderly.* New York: Oxford University Press.

Williams, J. S., & Engle, V. F. (1995). Staff evaluation of nursing home residents' competence. *Applied Nursing Research, 8*(1), 18–22.

Wunderlich, G. S., & Kohler, P. O. (Eds.). (2001). *Improving the quality of long-term care.* Washington, DC: National Academy Press.

Wunderlich, G. S., Sloan, F. A., & Davis, C. K. (1996). *Nursing staff in hospitals and nursing homes: Is it adequate?* Washington, DC: National Academy Press.

Xakellis, G. C., Frantz, R. A., Lewis, A., & Harvey, P. (1998). Cost-effectiveness of an intensive pressure ulcer prevention protocol in long-term care. *Advances in Wound Care, 11,* 22–29.

Yesavage, J. A., & Brink, T. L. (1983). Development and validation of a geriatric depression screening scale: A preliminary report. *Journal of Psychiatric Research, 17,* 37–49.

Zimmerman, D. R., Karon, S. L., Arling, G., Clark, B. R., Collins, T., Ross, R., & Sainfort, F. (1995). Development and testing of nursing home quality indicators. *Health Care Financing Review, 16*(4), 107–127.

Zinn, J. S., Brannon, D., & Weech, R. (1997). Quality improvement in nursing care facilities: Extent, impetus, and impact. *American Journal of Medical Quality, 12,* 51–61.

Index

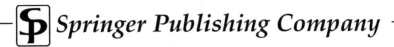

Community-Based Health

Research: *Issues and Methods*

Daniel S. Blumenthal, MD, MPH
Ralph J. DiClemente, PhD, Editors

"The editors of this book bring together in one place a description both of epidemiological methods and a discussion of community-level issues. It is a volume that will prove useful to those who wish to conduct contemporary community-based research." —from the Foreword by **David Satcher**, MD, PhD

This book identifies key concepts of successful community-based research beyond the aspect of location, including prevention focus, population-centered partnerships, multidisciplinary cooperation, and cultural competency. Lessons from the Tuskegee Syphilis Study and case studies on HIV/AIDS prevention and cardiovascular risk reduction illustrate the application of research methods with both positive and negative outcomes.

Contents:
• Foreword, *D. Satcher*

Part I: Issues
• Community-Based Research: An Introduction, *D.S. Blumenthal and E. Yancey*
• Assessing and Applying Community-Based Research, *C. Evans*
• Public Health Ethics and Community-Based Research: Lessons from the Tuskegee Syphilis Study, *B. Jenkins, C. Jones, and D.S. Blumenthal*
• The View from the Community, *A. Cruz, F. Murphy, N. Nyarko, and D.N.Y. Krall*

Part II: Methods
• Study Designs, Surveys, and Descriptive Studies, *N. Asal and L. Beebe*
• Survey Case Study: The Behavioral Risk Factor Surveillance System, *D. Holtzman*
• Qualitative Methods in Community-Based Research, *C. Sterk and K. Elifson*
• HIV/AIDS Prevention: Case Study in Qualitative Research, *K. Elifson and C. Sterk*
• Community Intervention Trials: Theoretical and Methodological Considerations, *R.J. DiClemente, R.A. Crosby, C. Sionean, and D. Holtgrave*
• Cardiovascular Risk Reduction Community Intervention Trials, *S.K. Davis*

2004   240pp   0-8261-2025-3   hard

536 Broadway, NY, NY 10012 • Fax: (212) 941-7842
Order Toll-Free: (877) 687-7476 • Order On-line: www.springerpub.com

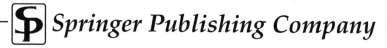 **Springer Publishing Company**

Diversity In Health Care Research
Strategies for Multisite, Multidisciplinary, and Multicultural Projects

Joellen W. Hawkins, RNC, PhD, FAAN
Lois A. Haggerty, RNC, PhD, Editors

The new gold standard in health care research is conducting studies that are truly representative of the general population—and not limited to a narrow range of cultural, gender, geographic, or socioeconomic groups. This book provides a how-to approach to planning, implementing, and conducting such studies. Especially valuable are case examples describing successful research projects that have taken on the "multi" approach.

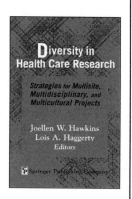

Partial Contents:

Part I: Strategies for Implementation

• Managing Multisite, Multidisciplinary, and Multi-Ethnic Research Projects, *N.W. Veeder*

• Facilitating Passage Through the Institutional Maze, *J.W. Hawkins, et al.*

• Using Research Assistants, *U.A. Kelly*

• International Multisite Studies, *L.J. Mayberry, et al.*

Part II: Lessons Learned from Specific Research Projects

• The Family Care Research Program: Testing the Efficacy of an Intervention Directed Toward Family Caregivers of Cancer Patients, *S.L. Kozachik, et al.*

• The Women's Health Initiative: Aspects of Management and Coordination, *B. Cochrane, B. Lund, S.Anderson, and R. Prentice*

Part III: In Conclusion

• Final Words, Many Voices, *J.W. Hawkins and L. Haggerty*

2003   264pp   0-8261-1814-3   *hard*

536 Broadway, NY, NY 10012 • Fax: (212) 941-7842

Order Toll-Free: (877) 687-7476 • Order On-line: www.springerpub.com